Positively PCOS

A story about infertility that led to the discovery of PCOS (Polycystic Ovary Syndrome)

By

Amy L. Hansen

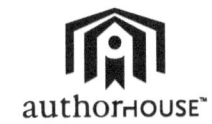

authorHOUSE™

1663 LIBERTY DRIVE, SUITE 200
BLOOMINGTON, INDIANA 47403
(800) 839-8640
WWW.AUTHORHOUSE.COM

First published by AuthorHouse 08/12/05

ISBN: 1-4208-1624-1 (sc)

Library of Congress Control Number: 2004099245

Printed in the United States of America
Bloomington, Indiana

This book is printed on acid-free paper.

I dedicate this book with love

to my children,

Erek and Emma,

and to the PCOS community.

Acknowledgements

I thank my husband, Ron, for being my true partner. I thank him for his love, understanding and support during treatment, and encouragement while pursuing this book project. We didn't know the depths that we'd have to go to for a family, but he hung in there with me with patience and compassion. I am also thankful for his quirky sense of humor; he can always make me laugh.

I thank my immediate and extended families for taking care of me when I was ill. Mom, I know that my treatments worried you on more than one occasion. Now that I am a mom, I know what it is like to worry about our children. Mom, I also thank you for your support on this book project and helping spread the word about PCOS.

I thank my good friend, Marty Ropog, for her brilliant insight while helping me edit this book. For without her, this may not have come to fruition. She is my literary goddess.

I thank my physicians, her staff and my midwife for truly connecting with me. You always made me feel as if I was your only patient, when I knew that that was not the case. The care and compassion you directed towards Ron and me will never be forgotten. We will carry you in our hearts forever.

I thank my dear girlfriends, Rose Duncan and Denise Kimerer, for always finding the time to listen when I needed to talk. I couldn't have made it through some of my roughest days without you. Thank you for not judging me and always accepting me.

My gratitude also goes to Lisa Garypie for coming up with the book's cover concept. The outreaching hands represent the help that I received from my support system, i.e. family, friends, and physicians. The butterflies are a symbol of the metamorphosis and change that happened to me during this process. According to **Animal Speak** by Ted Andrews, First Edition, 2005, "butterflies represent the process of transformation and the dance of joy. To Native Americans, the butterfly is a symbol of change, joy and color. When butterflies come into your life look at how much or how little joy is within your life. Lighten up. Look for change. Don't forget that all change is good."

Table of Contents

Reference to Inserts

Introduction

Neither Polycystic Ovary Syndrome (PCOS) nor Insulin Resistance (IR) is a death sentence. In most circumstances, they can be managed properly and brought under control. It does take knowledge, patience, determination, and physical and emotional strength.

This is the story of what started to be our pursuit to have a family. But it became much more. The diagnosis changed my life. I am not the same individual that I was when I began this quest. The road traveled was long, hard, painful and gratifying. But, in every way, worth the outcome!

The motive for communicating my story is knowledge. If one person walks away with a better understanding of PCOS, Insulin Resistance, in-vitro fertilization and other fertility issues, then my goal has been accomplished. I am not a medical doctor, but I am an experienced patient. I will not be able to provide the deepest level of understanding on these subjects, but I can relate my experiences. And sometimes, just that is helpful. I may sometimes come across as too technical or too basic in some of my explanations, but I wrote this in my own words, as I was experiencing it.

My hope is that, through these words, others like me will recognize their symptoms and inquire about medical treatment to prevent the possibility of other serious medical complications from developing. If this story allows someone to take comfort in comparing our struggles with theirs, or to help a loved one in need, it has served my purpose. I also hope this encourages people to become proactive about their medical care, and really open the lines of communication with their physician.

*So much has been written about infertility... diagnosis, causes, treatment, methods to achieve pregnancy, old wives tales, etc. But this story is different. As years went by without a pregnancy, I became frustrated with the treatments and this caused me to question many other things in my life that lead to something I wasn't prepared for. As I questioned my very purpose, changes began happening. My spirit and my soul would never be the same again. And for **that** I am grateful!*

In the beginning, I wasn't prepared or educated enough to take an active role in my diagnosis and treatment. But that quickly changed. I've come to believe that each person needs to take the responsibility to understand their own body's physiological needs. This means asking questions, doing your own research and, with the assistance of professionals, becoming an expert on your diagnosis and treatment.

My road was not an easy one to travel. It was full of emotional ups and downs; joys and heartaches, and physical pain. I've learned that the willpower of a woman who wants to achieve a successful pregnancy is unmatched by anything I have ever witnessed.

There are many struggles contained in this fight for family and health, and they are not always between husband and wife, or doctor and patient. These internal struggles can destroy your personal strength, hope and faith, but can ultimately change your life forever. My husband and I now look at the world through eyes that have been refocused and realigned.

It took 3½ years for me to become pregnant. To some couples, this may not seem like a very long time because others have tried longer, but to us it was an eternity. If you do the math, that's 42 opportunities to get pregnant for a normal-cycling woman. With the help of medications, we had 22 cycles over 42 months. We were finally successful on Cycle 22.

In the beginning of our quest to have a family, I thought I knew what it took. Looking back now, I see that I literally knew little. This is humbling. As my condition evolved, so did I. I grew into a well-informed, educated person and gained control of my life and body.

In the Beginning

Ron and I met when I was fifteen and he was eighteen. It was the summer of 1986. He was going to be a college freshman in the fall, and I was going to be a junior in high school. We dated for three years, became engaged when I was a freshman in college, and planned to be married two years later. Newly married in August 1991, I was just two months shy of turning twenty-one, and Ron was twenty-three. We were each working full-time during the day, going to school at night and working odd jobs on weekends as we steamed ahead with respective and shared goals.

When we married we agreed to wait five years to have children. We finished our degrees, had satisfying careers, and bought a house. Happily feathering our nest, we prepared for and dreamed of our children to come. Our story begins in the spring of 1996.

Let's Have a Baby

Spring 1996

Ron and I knew that we wanted to have a family someday. You know the dream: two parents, two kids, two cars, and a house with a picket fence. That didn't seem like such a farfetched dream. We were average, hard-working, middle-class newlyweds establishing our roots. It never crossed our minds that our experience would be any different from everyone else that we knew having children. We figured that once I stopped taking birth control pills (BCP's), within three months I'd be pregnant. This simple three month plan turned into a three-plus year process.

We were approaching our five-year anniversary, the timeframe we had set to begin our family, and I was excited about getting pregnant. My obstetrician/gynecologist (OB/GYN) advised me to discontinue taking the BCP's, and he recommended that I have another period on my own before trying to conceive.

I went off BCP's in mid-May 1996, and we began to use condoms as our alternative means of birth control. It didn't take long to notice that I wasn't cycling at all without BCP's. I did not have a period in June or July. On the one hand, of course, it was great during the summer months, but on the other hand, how was I supposed to get pregnant if I wasn't cycling? Not having a period wasn't a complete surprise to me, because before I went on BCP's at seventeen, I did not cycle regularly.

"The Lucky One"

My friends called me "The Lucky One". I probably had one or two menstrual cycles a year from the age of twelve until I went on BCP's at seventeen. At the time, I wasn't particularly concerned about this. As a matter of fact, I would guess that most young teens are not worried about missing menstrual cycles unless, of course, they are sexually active and worried about an accidental pregnancy.

When I began dating and contemplating a future family, thoughts crossed my mind that there must be something wrong with my female "parts," meaning uterus and ovaries. Maybe I didn't have all my "parts." If I didn't have all of my "parts," then how could I ever have children? At some level, I assumed that I did have my "parts," because as irregular as the cycles were, I did have at least <u>one</u> menstrual cycle a year. That had to count for something. But in my seventeen-year-old state of mind, "missing parts" still seemed reasonable, so I discussed this with my mom and she agreed to take me to a gynecologist for my first exam.

On our initial visit the doctor told us that most irregular cycles in adolescence are due to active lifestyles and developing hormones. He said that the inconsistently developing hormones can be attributed to emotional mood swings that are usually obvious in adolescents. I was a very active teen, but don't recall extreme emotional mood swings happening to me like they did to my friends. At the conclusion of my first visit, I was prescribed BCP's in order to regulate the cycles and hormone levels. I was seventeen and a senior in high school. The last thing I wanted was the reputation that went along with the other girls that were on BCP's. So I told no one, including my closest girlfriends.

So began my experience with birth control pills. They were great. I loved how scheduled and predictable my cycles were. Four days long, not much cramping, and none of those bad side effects like weight gain, acne, or heavy bleeding. These were some of the side effects they warned me to look for. There were several different prescription strengths that could be substituted, if needed.

Ten years later I found out that my treatment with BCP's at a young age probably saved me from the future development of endometriosis[1]. Over a prolonged period of time, this can lead to greater infertility difficulties and possibly pre-cancer conditions. Ron and I joked at the beginning of our fertility treatment that we could have saved $20 a month on BCP's for eight years. Now I know that those BCP's I took to prevent pregnancy probably prevented the development of endometriosis. I really was "The Lucky One."

---

[1]   Endometriosis – a condition in which endometrial (cells that line the uterus) tissue develops outside the uterus in the abdominal cavity.

The First Attempt

July 1996 – March 1997

In July 1996 we called my OB/GYN's office. I had not had a period since stopping BCP's two months earlier. The doctor told me that I probably would not have regular periods because of my history before BCP's. He suggested waiting until the end of the summer, then trying a pregnancy test. He told me that even though I didn't have regular menses, I could possibly still ovulate and conceive. Ron and I agreed to try and we discontinued the use of contraception. We were planning to celebrate our five-year anniversary in August by taking a cruise to Mexico. Wouldn't it be lovely to conceive our child on the trip!

The Monday we returned, I was in the doctor's office taking a urine pregnancy test. As I exited the restroom, the billing clerk actually congratulated me.

"I understand that you have good news?" she said.

"Um, not that I'm aware of, but that is why I'm here." was my response.

Evidently, in their practice, when a patient gets pregnant, the medical chart gets re-categorized and filed with the "pregnant" charts. My doctor predicted that we were pregnant because I did not have any cycles all summer.

Well, guess what. The pregnancy test was negative. This was the beginning of one hell-of-a-long emotionally winding road. Although I didn't really think that I was pregnant, it was kind of neat thinking that I could have been. But this was my first negative pregnancy test. At this point, I never could have imagined how many times I would be peeing on a stick or into a small Dixie cup, eagerly waiting for the colors to change.

The doctor prescribed a pill for me called Provera™. Provera™ (also available as Cycrin™) is a brand name for medroxyprogesterone acetate (MPA). It is a progestin, not progesterone[2]. Progestins are typically used to bring on a period, and supplemental progesterone is given on the premise that there is an inadequate amount of natural progesterone to support a pregnancy. My doctor explained that by inducing a period, we would have a good starting point. The instructions were to take Provera™ for 10 days, and within a few days of finishing the prescription I should start my period. He then instructed us to have unprotected intercourse as often as every other day for two months. "Well, that might likely kill me," I joked, but I was sure that my husband would be delighted.

At that time, I didn't even know the full stages of menstruation. I remember asking what the most fertile days in the cycle were. He told me that an egg is typically released from the ovary approximately 14 days after the first full day of full bleeding. He supported his instructions with the explanation that it takes most normally-cycling people six months to conceive. He told me that he didn't want

---

[2] The progestin "matures" the uterine lining and the withdrawal from the medication is what induces a period, as opposed to progesterone which is the hormone naturally produced by the corpus luteum following ovulation to create a lush environment in the uterine lining that is receptive to pregnancy.

to get too aggressive right then with advanced testing or treatment even though I wasn't cycling regularly. He said that it didn't mean that I couldn't or wouldn't get pregnant, "happens all the time." The note in my medical chart for that visit read "may need Clomid, and start Provera for 10 days, watch for 2 months." [3]

I had a Provera-induced period in September. When that was over, Ron and I were like machines. We tried as hard as we could to keep up the every-other-day schedule. We especially stepped it up around cycle days 12-16, just to make sure we captured one of my eggs.

No period in October. I called my doctor and was told to keep trying for two more months, and call in January if still no success. The plan then would be to try Clomid™.

By November, two of our friends had their first babies. One couple got pregnant on the second try and the other couple wasn't even trying. They each had wonderful little healthy babies. At this point we were very excited for them and we were pretty excited for us too because we were sure we would be announcing a pregnancy soon.

It was now December and it had been four months since our last pregnancy test. I still had not cycled since September - 101 days. I called the doctor's office again and was told that we were probably pregnant. So off I went to the OB/GYN for another urine test. I practiced my aim into the cup and, with big hopes, gave the sample to the nurse. Wait, wait, and wait. Ten minutes is an eternity. Do you know how many baby thoughts you can have in ten minutes? The due date, girl names, boy names. Well, they were short-lived thoughts; the test was a big, fat, Negative.

He gave me Provera™ once again to induce a cycle, and he said to call him when I started my period; he would then prescribe medication that would help me ovulate. Hurray! Something to make me ovulate! Now we were getting somewhere. We were getting assistance with "fertility" medication and it wouldn't take long now.

At that time, he also ordered a semen analysis for Ron, just so we could make sure that there weren't any male factors inhibiting our ability to conceive. For a semen analysis, the specimen must be collected in a sterile cup and kept warm while being transported to the lab. There are four items that are tested and noted. The first is the overall volume. The normal volume of semen is between 2 and 5 milliliters (ml). Some factors that can affect volume are the number of times of recent ejaculation, blockages and different medications. Second, they assess sperm count; the actual number of sperm per ml of semen. The count can vary widely, but any number greater than 20 million per ml is considered normal and there is no such thing as too many. Anything fewer than 20 million per ml of semen may indicate something to look into. They would then also assess total sperm count, versus per ml. The third test is on sperm motility, or

---

[3]   When I went back to do research for this book, I gathered my old medical chart comments and have included some of them throughout the book.

the movement of the sperm. Our lab report stated that normal motility can be anywhere from 40–70%. This means that 40-70% of the sperm are mobile. And the fourth test is for morphology. Morphology refers to the shape of the sperm. They will report the percentage of normal vs. abnormal morphology. Our lab results did not state what the normal morphology limits were. Sperm develop in many different shapes. Although some are formed with two "heads", or two tails, a sperm with one head and one long tail are considered normal. Ron's sperm test results were listed as 2.4 ml in volume, 120.6 million/ml count, 67% motility and morphology showed 49% normal and 51% abnormal. The lab we used reported normal motility between 80 – 90%, so during the time of this test Ron's sperm had low motility. My OB/GYN prescribed an antibiotic for him, predicting that he may have had an infection. He explained that sometimes certain infections can affect sperm production, but he didn't tell us much more than that. Ron took an oral antibiotic for about a week.

I started my Provera-induced period on January 1, 1997.[4]

My OB/GYN called in the prescription for Clomid™, one 50 mg tablet each day for five days. Clomid™ is typically the first step in any fertility therapy. Compared to other forms of treatment, it is a relatively low-cost medication, and 70% of woman treated are pregnant within the first three months of using Clomid™.

Clomid™ (clomiphene citrate) is not a hormone, but a synthetic, estrogen-like substance. Its function is to induce ovulation by fooling the body into believing that its estrogen level is low. Therefore, the hypothalamus produces greater levels of gonadotropin releasing hormone (GnRH), which triggers the increased production of luteinizing hormone (LH) and follicle stimulating hormone (FSH) from the pituitary gland. These increases in hormones cause the ovary to release an egg. Other brand names for clomiphene citrate are Serophene™ and Milophene™.

The hormones, GnRH, LH and FSH will be mentioned many times throughout this story. In order to increase my understanding of the production and interaction of these hormones, I eventually developed a simplified graph diagram that depicts the hormone flow. This is found in **Appendix A**. I did not develop this little "cheat sheet" of hormonal flow until my later treatment years, but it may prove to be useful as a reference. At this early point of treatment, I had never even heard of these hormones, let alone know how they affected my reproductive cycle.

Okay, so far this seems pretty easy, but I had heard terrible stories from people that had to take "fertility" medication. Most stories were about the awful side effects and great emotional distress they endured. I wasn't too sure what to expect.

I read the warning labels on the medication to Ron. It warned that the possible side effects of Clomid™ were hot flashes, nausea, vomiting, breast tenderness, dizziness, lightheadedness, headache, or mood changes, and cautioned that using

---

4   In order to keep them organized throughout the story, I number all of my cycles starting with this one. This was cycle #1. I will also refer many times to my Cycle Day. The first full day of bleeding is Cycle Day 1 (CD 1).

this medicine might result in multiple gestation (twins, triplets, etc.). The caution on multiple gestation stood out the most dramatically to us. We were thinking, "whew boy, the possibility of more than one." But I didn't worry. I just knew that we were in the home stretch now. A couple of tries with this Clomid™, and we would be well on our way to parenthood.

Like the lead detective in an investigation, I began asking everyone at work about Clomid™. What had they heard, or maybe anyone that had used it and what their experiences were. One woman co-worker said that it worked for a friend of hers on the second cycle. This reinforced my hope that it wasn't going to be long now.

Parenthood, here we come! I quickly had visions of Ron and me pushing a child on a swing, running through a pile of crispy fall leaves, and building our first snowman. It was all coming together.

After I finished the Clomid™, we were on CD 6. The doctor told us that I could ovulate anywhere between cycle days 12 and 19. We were told that it was best to have intercourse every other day during that time period. Sperm can live anywhere from 24-48 hours in the female reproductive tract, so we had intercourse on CD 13, 16 and 19.

Without a period by CD 30, we were pretty happy. This was probably it. We couldn't wait to get the good news. I went in on February 4 for my urine pregnancy test. Same procedure: hold cup, aim, fire, clean hands, turn in sample and WAIT. Let's see, what nursery theme would we choose, would it be a boy or girl, what if it is a boy AND a girl?

Well, we would have to keep on dreaming because the test was another Big Fat Negative. This was about the time that we should have bought stock in the companies that make home pregnancy test kits (HPT's). I estimate that over the 3-year ordeal I bought approximately twenty-seven HPT's, in addition to the urine tests that I took at the OB/GYN's office.

I went home from the doctor's office with instructions to call them when my period started. Since I was on CD 30, it should have been at any time.

Cycle # 2 thru 5

March – August 1997

My period did not come until **71 days** later when we were on vacation at Disney World. I have to say that throughout this story there seems to be a pattern of my period starting during every single vacation. If my periods weren't consistent, I could at least count on them coming while traveling.

I have often wondered if emotional distress can trigger hormonal changes that can induce a menstrual cycle. I do not know if there is a scientific answer, but the correlation in my situation was uncanny. I became very upset one evening while on vacation and, BOOM, the very next morning I was greeted with my long-awaited period.

After we returned from vacation, I called the doctor to give him the news about my cycle. He asked me to come in for some blood work. I did not pay any attention to the results of that blood work until researching this book. At the time of the blood test I did not even ask about the results, but I'm not sure that I would have understood them anyway. The analysis showed my FsH level at 7.1 and my TsH level at 2.43, both of which were normal. At the time, I didn't know what the tests or the results meant. I have since read that the FsH blood test is very difficult to interpret unless you know the exact length of your cycle. My prolactin level was also tested and came back at 10; the only thing I knew about prolactin is that it could inhibit ovulation. Prolactin is the hormone that is released in the body when a woman is breastfeeding. It is the body's natural way of inhibiting another pregnancy while breastfeeding.

It was at that visit that the OB/GYN suggested I start taking my basal body temperature (BBT) readings and plotting them. This requires taking your temperature BEFORE getting out of bed in the morning, writing it down, and charting it on a graph to see the pattern. Before this exercise was explained to me, I did not actually know that body temperature spikes during ovulation, or when an egg is released. It doesn't rise dramatically like five degrees or anything, but possibly one-half to one degree. I started charting my BBT on March 31. Since we were already a week into cycle # 2, the doctor said to call when cycle # 3 started so we could start Clomid™ again. So cycle # 2 had no Clomid™, but I was measuring my BBT.

This was the beginning of any kind of record-keeping. Up to that point, I had only been keeping track of the days that I started a cycle and when I went to the doctor. My advice to you is to keep a journal or log of everything that goes on with your individual treatment plan. A copy of the log that I created and used is in **Appendix B**. Items to include should be date, cycle day, medications, HPT, doctor visits, BBT reading, blood tests, intercourse, feelings, and observations.

The BBT process was groundbreaking for us. When I charted my BBT measurements, it demonstrated an irregular pattern to my temperature movements. There was no temperature peak (which typically indicates ovulation); my BBT was all over the board, which indicated the most likely conclusion of NO ovulation

7

at all, or "anovulation." I wish that I had known then what I know now. As a patient with a history of anovulation, this should have been our first exercise a year previous. It would have at least saved us some time and frustration over the previous ten months. I have my BBT charts listed in **Appendix C**.

As CD 30 approached I hoped with all my might that I would not start my period. That could only mean one thing to us …pregnant. I took an HPT on CD 30 and waited the agonizing ten minutes only to find out that there was no blue line on the stick. Boy, were we getting used to that. I was beginning to doubt that HPT's ever worked at all.

I called the OB/GYN as CD 44 approached and explained what was going on. I had not started another period yet, and my BBT readings had absolutely no pattern to them. I made an appointment and went in to see him in early May. During my visit I took another urine pregnancy test. He just wanted to make sure the result was negative, before we proceeded. Of course, it was!

We didn't induce a period this time with Provera™. We just started another round of Clomid™. And that ended cycle # 2 and launched cycle # 3.

This time he doubled the dosage of Clomid™ to 100 mg. The pharmacy gave me the generic for Clomid™ called Serophene™. I took the Serophene™ for five days. We watched the BBT chart very closely this time and had intercourse four times in the four days around ovulation. We thought our chances seemed pretty good. We could see the temperature change on our chart this time. The BBT results improved dramatically with the double dosage this time.

When CD 30 came and went, we didn't even get our hopes up this time. I took an HPT and the result was negative. So I called the OB/GYN office to report in. Another urine pregnancy test at the doctor's office verified it was negative. I was given another prescription for 100 mg of Clomid™, and again the pharmacy filled it with Serophene™. This ended cycle # 3 and launched cycle # 4.

Ron and I had intercourse four more times in the four days around ovulation. We always tried so hard to keep our sense of humor throughout this ordeal. I would try to keep things in perspective, but this was very draining for me emotionally. If I only knew then what I know now. We still had so far to go!

It was about this time that my sister, Jen, and I took a girl trip to Myrtle Beach. That trip gave us an opportunity to catch up because we didn't get to see each other very often. I confided in her and told her about my infertility treatment and that we would get the results upon my return from the trip. My sister mentioned that our mom had wanted her to attempt to find out if we were trying for a baby yet. I told her that she could tell Mom that we were trying, but nothing more than that. I didn't want my mom to be worried about Ron and me.

At that point, only my sister knew of our difficulties. Our family and friends knew that we were trying, but had no idea the degree of difficulty we were having. I did not want to divulge everything because people always ask how things are going. I am sure everyone is genuinely concerned, but their inquiries are a constant reminder of the frustration of treatment. So our choice was to keep a lid on things until we could announce our good news.

We even had people ask if we decided NOT to have a family or why we didn't have any children yet. One person actually told us they heard that we didn't want to have any children because we wanted to keep our money to ourselves. How about that for a rude comment! I keep trying to tell myself that it takes all kinds of people to make the world go 'round. And some people are just plain old hurtful to others. But Ron and I are strong individuals, and we are even stronger together. We just let the comments roll off of our backs.

We do have some very close friends that could probably sense that we were having difficulties, but they never asked. I appreciated that. At the time I just struggled terribly with discussing this with anyone. I was always hopeful that the next cycle would be the successful one. Most of our friends had at least one child by then, and Ron and I always looked forward to visiting and playing with the babies. I know some people that suffer from infertility avoid being around children, or parents with children for that matter, because the pain is so bitter. But I just never felt jealousy or anger towards our friends. They were not to blame for our unfortunate situation, and admitting this is half the battle. However, this type of an ordeal can sometimes dissolve friendships that have survived many other obstacles. Not necessarily because the adults have changed who they are, but friends that have children are changed because they live in a world of children's activities, i.e. birthday parties, theme parks, zoo, school, sports, etc. and the likelihood of having things in common is reduced.

After my sister and I returned from our beach vacation, I had a renewed sense of belief that everything was going to work out that cycle. We waited as the days slowly went by. Then something very surprising happened - I started my period on CD 29. We didn't even make it to CD 30 for the pregnancy test.

That launched cycle # 5 in early July. I reported in with the OB/GYN office and they prescribed the last round of 100 mg Clomid™ again. The note in my OB/GYN's file said "try one more month of Clomid, to Smith[5] if no success." Once again the pharmacy gave me the Clomid™ generic, Serophene™, and I took it for five days. Ron and I followed our scheduled intercourse sessions once a day for the days of my predicted ovulation. But all efforts failed. I started my period on CD 34.

---

[5]   Name has been changed for privacy.

Cycle # 6 and 7 – Referral to Specialist

August – October 1997

Cycle # 6 came in early August. Now remember that it had been sixteen months since Ron and I consciously decided to try to have a baby. Over that time I only had <u>six</u> cycles to work with, not sixteen. Since the previous three cycles with Clomid™ and charting my BBT did not result in a pregnancy, we were referred to Dr. Smith, a reproductive endocrinologist (RE). A reproductive endocrinologist is a physician that specializes in the treatment of disorders of the reproductive hormonal system and reproductive organs in men and women.

However, when I called to set up an appointment at Dr. Smith's office, the waiting period for a new patient with consultation was six weeks to three months. I just about flipped out! More waiting. The person on the phone asked if we had any objection to seeing Dr. Gold; she would be available sooner than Dr. Smith. Since we didn't know either one at the time, we didn't have a problem with it. We were able to get an appointment within six weeks to see Dr. Gold. Our appointment was in late September. It seemed like an eternity away.

By now I had developed an overwhelming feeling of helplessness, like my body was out of my control and there was nothing I could do about it. I could control every other factor in my life, but not this one. It made me angry. It just wasn't fair! We worked so hard for everything else we had achieved, why couldn't we have a baby? It made me doubt my abilities, and who I was. This was not normal for me…I am sure some of these feelings were generated because I have a classic type A personality. Type A personality has been described as people who are always on the move, have a strong sense of urgency, often sit on the edge of their seats, literally, check their watches more frequently, are often obsessed with their work, extremely competitive, want to get things done and they will do almost anything to accomplish their goals. They tend to become aggressive, impatient, and irritable to anyone or anything that interferes with their work. Sounds delightful doesn't it? The feeling of being out of control is very debilitating to me.

Then of course I turned the blame to a higher being. Maybe there was some underlying reason God did not want us to have children. I didn't think we were undeserving. But maybe He knew something we didn't. What had we done? Why us? These questions went through my mind, as I am sure it does with other infertile couples.

Just a week before our RE consultation, I went away for the weekend with my girlfriends. And as I should have predicted, I started cycle # 7 on the trip.

Ron and I went to our initial fertility consultation not really knowing what to expect. The RE had requested my files from my OB/GYN and she asked us to describe our history to her. After we spoke about our past treatment, she went on to describe many things. She began with an explanation of the hormonal changes that have to be present to initiate the reproductive process in a woman. To my surprise, she explained that hormonal signals that come from the pituitary gland are what regulate the reproductive organs. All of this new information was very fascinating, but at the same time very overwhelming.

During her explanation, she wrote down key words on a tablet of paper. It was totally *Greek* to me. I asked if I could keep this paper for reference. When I read this piece of paper now, it seems like the "holy grail." The following key words were taken from her notes:

- Insulin Resistance – Receptor on ovary, Fasting insulin/glucose.
- Ovulation Induction – Clomid - recruitment [of eggs] plus Fertinex (injectible "Food for Eggs"), 15% twins possibility.
- Ovulation Induction with full FSH has 20% possibility of twins, 5% chance of triplets.
- Intrauterine Insemination.
- In Vitro Fertilization. Profasi (HcG) - 1.) Releases eggs, 2.) Mature DNA, 3.) Prepares endometrium lining.

She said that her practice treats people with symptoms similar to ours, many of whom have achieved successful results. She told us that there was no reason why we should give up hope for a family yet. Whew, we both breathed a sigh of relief. She gave Ron and me a reason to finally smile again.

Dr. Gold described and drew a "normal" female reproductive cycle. This visual description helped me to gain a better understanding of what needed to take place in order to achieve a pregnancy.

She prescribed an entire series of medications and explained what each one would do. Each medication was a substitute for a hormone that should be produced by my body naturally, but for some reason was not. The medications prescribed were Provera™, Clomid™, Fertinex™, Profasi™, and prenatal vitamins. I was familiar with Provera™, Clomid™, and prenatal vitamins, but the others were new to me. I knew that Provera™ makes your period start, and Clomid™ would trigger ovulation. Fertinex™ was described as "food" to make the eggs grow, and Profasi™ would release the eggs when they were done "growing."

Fertinex™ is a brand name for a gonadotropin[6] injection. It simulates the hormone, follicle stimulating hormone, or FsH that is normally produced by the pituitary gland. It comes in a vial as dry powder and must be mixed with the accompanying vial of saline before injecting. Profasi™ is a brand name for human chorionic gonadotropin (hCG) injection. Biologically, hCG is identical to luteinizing hormone (LH) and causes the same response, which is to "release" the eggs from the ovaries. According to <u>PCOS: The Hidden Epidemic</u> (p. 385), hCG can be equally substituted for LH in therapy.

These are important terms to remember because I refer to these many times as the story progresses.

We did not walk away with a "diagnosis" for my infertility that day. But we did walk away with a sense of accomplishment and regained hope. As long as I had hope, I had the desire to fight the battle.

---

[6] Gonadotropins – Hormones (FSH, LH) produced by the pituitary gland to stimulate the ovaries to produce eggs.

I was very excited to start the new medication regime. Once again, I thought this was even a bigger deal than our previous treatments. We were using injectibles now. This was serious business. I truly believed that I'd be pregnant within two cycles. We were very optimistic!

Before we left the office, the nurse trained Ron and me how to load the syringe with the medication from the vials. She also gave us a training video that we could watch at home if we needed help. She showed us where to administer the shots for each type of medication. The subcutaneous, or "under the skin," shots could go in my thigh, the belly area, or in the flabby part of my upper arm. The needles are not that long and just need to go under the skin. The administration of an intramuscular, or "in the muscle," shot was a little more specific. The needle length was about 1½ inches and needed to be administered into a muscle. The easiest location for this shot was in the rear-end.

The other noticeable difference between my intramuscular and subcutaneous shots was the needle gauge. Needle gauge refers to the thickness of the actual needle. The smaller the gauge number, the thicker the needle. And vice versa, needles with a larger gauge number have a thinner needle. The thicker needles (smaller gauge numbers) can sometimes sting a little more than the thinner ones.

During our initial consultation, I was on CD 7. Dr. Gold instructed me to come back for a pregnancy blood test on CD 28. If the test came back negative, then I would need to start taking one Provera™ a day for seven days. The withdrawal of the Provera™ would start a period, which I already knew. Once the new cycle began, I would need to start taking a double dose of 100 mg of Clomid™ on CD 3-7, then one ampule (amp) of Fertinex™ a day on each cycle day 8-11, followed up by a transvaginal ultrasound[7]. WOW! All that for just one cycle. I was impressed.

My blood test on CD 28 was negative. This was my first <u>blood</u> test for pregnancy results. I never took another urine test at the doctor's, only the HPT's that I did at home. During our first consultation in September, the doctor had requested that I fast before going for my pregnancy blood test on CD 28 because she also wanted to check my fasting insulin and fasting glucose levels. The insulin came back at a 12.5 and the glucose came back at 85. At the time, I had <u>no idea</u> what these numbers meant, and furthermore, couldn't understand why she would want blood sugar levels drawn. I remember when the results came back, my RE told me that they were OK numbers. I didn't question it or research it any further again until much later.

---

[7] Transvaginal ultrasound – A wand (transducer) is inserted into the vagina in order to examine the ovaries and uterus via ultrasound.

Cycle # 8

October - November 1997

I started Provera™ the day of the negative pregnancy test and cycle # 8 started within days. I followed up with all the other medications as instructed.

This would be our first cycle that required administration of injectible medication at home. We were so careful to follow the directions precisely. Our bathroom counter looked like a pharmacy to me, with so many supplies and medications. We had alcohol swabs, syringes, cotton balls, and four different medications. The Fertinex™ came with two vials; one vial filled with saline that was to be mixed with the other vial that held the dry powdered medication. Ron and I alternated filling the syringes each day, so that we each got practice. Even though we both took turns filling the syringe, Ron always administered the shot in the side of my thigh, alternating legs each day. The thigh area was the most comfortable for me. My thighs had more fat than my arms. I thought the belly or arm sounded more painful. During these early cycles, Ron injected all of the shots. At the time, I couldn't tolerate self-administering. I felt woozy as soon as the needle got close to my skin.

Ron really helped ease my tensions when we did injections by joking around and making me laugh. I was sure that he just loved the opportunity to inject me with a needle. He told me how cool it was. Even though infertility is often a very emotional ordeal, I would recommend trying to keep a sense of humor during the treatment cycles. I know it isn't easy for everyone, but laughing usually lifted my spirits a little bit, and Ron has a knack for saying just the right thing.

We also made it a practice to go to my doctor appointments together, when possible. I didn't want him to be left out of the learning curve. When it wasn't possible to go together, I explained everything to him when I got home. This kept us both educated and in this together. Ron now claims that he knows more about the female reproductive process now than he would have learned in an entire lifetime. Each spouse/partner is different though, and may experience different feelings during the treatment stages than the patient does. Fortunately, we were able to keep our hopes high and spirits light for each treatment. We were also very fortunate that this ordeal brought our relationship closer than ever, rather than farther apart. I really counted on him for so many things, but what stood out the most was emotional support. When I needed to vent, he would listen. Support is such an important part of the battle. Support comes in many forms, and if a spouse/partner is not able to fill the void completely, there are many alternatives, i.e. infertility website bulletin boards, support groups at clinics and counselors. This is very important to consider.

In early November, I had my first transvaginal ultrasound. It wasn't difficult at all. The speculum used for a Pap[8] smear was more uncomfortable.

---

[8]   Pap smear - Common name of a procedure developed by George Papanicolaou (1883-1962) to detect abnormal cells in the cervix.

The ultrasound machine has a monitor and keyboard on it, and the hand-held sonogram wand is connected by a cable. First, the nurse asked me to empty my bladder in the restroom, because a full bladder can block the view of the ovaries. Then the doctor inserted the wand into my vagina and looked at the uterine lining and ovaries.

My doctor explained what she was looking for as she went along. She pointed out the endometrium lining, measured it, and then went to view each ovary. She measured the diameter of each "follicle" on the left ovary, then moved to the right ovary. While she was measuring the follicles, the nurse was writing the measurements down in my chart. The left ovary had two follicles measuring 8 mm each, and the right ovary had follicles measuring 8½ , 8, and many less than 6 mm. They said that the growth of the follicles would be monitored and tracked against the amount of medication I was taking. At that point, I didn't even understand what "follicles" were and didn't really know what she was trying to achieve.

My doctor told me to increase to 2 amps of Fertinex™ that evening and the following night, then come back on the third day for another ultrasound. Before I left the doctor's office, the nurse called in the prescription for 4 more amps of Fertinex™ to the hospital pharmacy. This was very helpful for two reasons. First, I was on my lunch hour for the office visit and the pharmacy was on the way out. Secondly the hospital pharmacy was most likely going to have the Fertinex™ in stock immediately. I soon discovered that the pharmacy near my home had a hard time getting the injectables quickly. This was unacceptable when I needed them for immediate use.

Before we left that visit, Ron and I were also taught how to administer double doses of the Fertinex™ from the ampules. We injected 2 amps per night for two nights and were back in the office two days later for the ultrasound.

Dr. Gold and her nurse, Sandy, performed the ultrasound and quickly determined that the follicles had not grown at all in the last two days. Sandy left the room and Dr. Gold told me that we might have better luck next time. I was dumbfounded. I had it set in my mind that this was going to work. Remember? Two cycles and we were going to be pregnant. This prompted me to ask questions. What happened? Why does the cycle need to be terminated? What are you looking for to make it a "good" cycle? What size do these follicles have to be?

She began by explaining that treatment is unique to each person. We were trying to achieve the growth and maturity of an egg. One egg[9] is held within each of the follicles, which look like blisters on the ovary. A normal cycle will produce just **one** follicle a month and release an egg. In addition to an egg, there is fluid within these follicles. Once the egg matures, the matured egg needs to release from the follicle, get fertilized, travel down the fallopian tube, and implant in the uterus. The eggs needs follicle stimulating hormone (FsH) in order to grow. That is what the Fertinex™ is providing to them. Under normal circumstances, your pituitary gland regulates the release of this FsH. She said that my body weight

---

[9]   Also called an oocyte.

(approximately 140 pounds) did not lead her to believe that I would require a higher dose of the Fertinex™, one amp for six days. However, my ovaries did not react as well as she would have thought. Why? We did not know yet. Each person has completely different tolerances and reactions to every medication. She said that our goal was to get the follicles on my ovary to approximately 18-20 mm in diameter[10]. Follicles that are much smaller than 14 mm are sometimes not large enough to create a matured egg. Therefore, my cycle was canceled because the follicles were too small. So my doctor gave me a new prescription for 2 amps per day of Fertinex™ for the next cycle. She also asked me to save the Profasi™ that she prescribed earlier for the next cycle.

This was the first indication of having evidence of polycystic ovaries, which eventually led to the diagnosis of Polycystic Ovary Syndrome. At the time, I did not understand the terminology or the diagnosis. I didn't even realize that my symptoms had a name.

I knew more now than when I went in that day. I left excited about the new information we shared, but disappointed to have to begin waiting again. I had to wait for my period to start before I could start my new series of medications.

The waiting game for this cycle went by rather quickly, because I had a business trip to San Francisco that preoccupied me. Although, the due date for my period came and went without the start of my cycle.

Cycle # 8 - Summary

CD 3	100 mg Clomid™
CD 4	100 mg Clomid™
CD 5	100 mg Clomid™
CD 6	100 mg Clomid™
CD 7	100 mg Clomid™
CD 8	1 amp Fertinex™
CD 9	1 amp Fertinex™
CD 10	1 amp Fertinex™
CD 11	1 amp Fertinex™, ultrasound
CD 12	2 amps Fertinex™
CD 13	2 amps Fertinex™, ultrasound, Stop Cycle

---

[10] According to PCOS: The Hidden Epidemic, "the preovulatory follicle of a natural cycle is usually ovulated at about 20-23 mm. With Clomid™ the follicles may grow larger, around 24-30 mm. While on gonadotropins they are smaller, about 18-22 mm at time of ovulation." Page 78.

Cycle # 9

November – December 1997

I called my doctor's office to tell them that I had no sign of starting my cycle. They called in a new prescription with a new set of instructions. In mid-November, I started Provera™ for six days. Within nine days, I started cycle # 9. My doctor tripled the dosage of Clomid™ to 150 mg for CD 5-9, then 2 amps of Fertinex™ on CD 9-13, followed up by an ultrasound on CD 14. Single and double doses of Clomid™ didn't seem to affect me that much, but triple doses just about put me over the edge. Can you say MOOD SWINGS? I was also experiencing a lot of dizziness. I was a bit worried when I drove my car. Luckily, I never got dizzy while driving. It was a little strange sometimes. I was experiencing all of this commotion behind the scenes of my daily responsibilities.

My first ultrasound showed that my ovaries produced much better results than the last time. I had at least one follicle on the left ovary at 13 mm and two on the right at 13 and 12½ mm. I asked how many follicles we were trying to get. She said that that was difficult to answer. The more follicles you have reaching maturity (18-20 mm), the higher the number of eggs that could be released. This could result in multiple births, and this is a concern. Multiple births have the possibility of greater risks concerning complications to the mother and/or the possibility of multiple fetuses. One side effect to the patient is ovarian hyperstimulation syndrome (OHSS), a very dangerous condition in which the ovaries become over-stimulated. This syndrome is described in further detail in the chapter on Cycle # 17. Each person reacts differently to the medication; this is why it is so hard to develop the perfect recipe of medication to prescribe for each individual. An RE needs to be cautious with the prescribed level of medication for each patient. In my case, a standard medication protocol (single doses) for my body size and weight was not effective thus far.

I was given instructions to take 2½ amps of Fertinex™ the next two days, then come in for another ultrasound. I went back again two days later. The left ovary had a follicle measuring 17 mm and the right had ones that measured 17 and a 19 mm. Looking good! My nurse asked if I felt "full," like after I'd eaten dinner. I said "yes, and it's a little painful and tender in my belly area also." They said that that is a result from the number of follicles developing on the ovaries. The ovaries are enlarged and the cause for my abdominal swelling. My doctor prescribed Percocet for the pain. The Percocet was so strong; I was finally able to sleep for hours without the pain waking me up.

My doctor's instructions were to take 1 more amp of Fertinex™ that night, and administer the one vial of Profasi™ (10 k) the following evening. Then 32-36 hours after the administration of the Profasi™, we were to have intercourse. That was our first intramuscular shot at home on our own. They also recommended that we have intercourse once every day or every other day after that. The doctor recommended that we not have intercourse now until after the Profasi™ shot.

It didn't take long to get used to the subcutaneous shots. During our previous doctor visit, Ron and I were taught where to administer the intramuscular Profasi™ shot. He needed to put his right hand on my right hip with his thumb on my pelvic bone and fingers on my butt pointed down toward the floor.[11] The area of my butt that the tips of his fingers were touching was where the needle needed to go. It was the upper corner of my butt cheek. I liked to lean on the bathroom counter and stand on the opposite leg of the butt cheek that he was going to poke. This practice made the shot a little less painful for me; not painless, just less painful.

During our scheduled intercourse, one thing became evident very quickly. I was very uncomfortable. My ovaries were so swollen from the growth of the follicles that it caused my abdomen to be tender and painful. This condition did not lend itself well to comfortable intercourse. I could not stand ANY pressure in my belly area, so that meant Ron had to be a little extra sensitive to make it more comfortable for me. You'd think that conceiving a baby would be one of the most wonderful experiences in the world, but our experience up to this point had been a little different than most. We will never be able to tell our child that he/she was not planned.

We waited quietly through the Christmas holiday season, keeping our thoughts positive for conception. The ovary response was so encouraging, I just knew we would have good news to share with the family soon.

Ultimately, our sad news arrived on December 28, 1997 with the onset of cycle # 10. It didn't work. It didn't seem as if anything would EVER work for us. I had such high hopes for this cycle. Everything looked so good. I had quite a hard time dealing with the results. When I called the doctor's office to report the bad news, they asked me if I wanted to take a break before starting another cycle. I am sure they sensed my disappointment. I instinctively said no. I needed to proceed. So they called in another round of medications. All the same as before, except the Provera™. I had already started my period and wouldn't need it.

There were some other sad and difficult events in our family at the same time we received the negative pregnancy news. A very young friend of ours died very suddenly on Christmas Eve, leaving a husband and a three-month old daughter. All of this, combined with the personal infertility struggle that no one else knew about, took a pretty good toll on me. I was emotionally and physically drained and heartbroken . Under these circumstances, I contracted a terrible cold.

I fell into a deep feeling of helplessness very quickly. I was depressed, angry, frustrated, and feeling isolated. On top of all that, I was also just plain sick. It was one of the lowest points I can remember ever being in. How can this be happening? Why couldn't we get pregnant? Why was God doing this to us? Why was it so easy for everybody else? What had we done to deserve this? If this treatment worked for other people, why wasn't it working for us?

I affirmed my feelings of anger and resentment by rehashing these questions all day long and closed myself off from other people. I was so angry that this was

---

[11]   There is no significance to using the right side, you can use the left also.

happening to us. Why not pick on someone else? As far as I was concerned, we didn't do anything to deserve this (*like this is something people deserve*).

And then there was the money issue. We were using our savings for treatments, which now seemed like a waste. I was empty emotionally, physically, spiritually. And now we would be slowly drained financially. That was like the icing on the cake.

In addition, we felt such isolation when we secretly mourned each and every negative result. As if we had lost just one more piece of our future. It made everything so uncertain; uncertain that we would ever have a family, uncertain that we could afford more treatment, uncertain that we'd survive this struggle. We so desperately wanted to share parenthood together. The more I worried about this uncertainty, the more I cried and the sadder I got.

Even though I was at this low point in my life, I still insisted upon continuing treatment.

Cycle # 9 - Summary	
CD 5	150 mg Clomid™
CD 6	150 mg Clomid™
CD 7	150 mg Clomid™
CD 8	150 mg Clomid™
CD 9	150 mg Clomid™
CD 10	2 amps Fertinex™
CD 11	2 amps Fertinex™
CD 12	2 amps Fertinex™
CD 13	2 amps Fertinex™, ultrasound
CD 14	2½ amps Fertinex™
CD 15	2½ amps Fertinex™, ultrasound
CD 16	1 amp Fertinex™
CD 17	10k unit Profasi™ (HcG)

Cycle # 10 thru 12

December 1997 – May 1998

For the new cycle, Dr. Gold wanted me to take triple doses of Clomid™ on CD 3-7, then 2 amps of Fertinex™ a day on CD 6-11, and return to check my progress by ultrasound.

I started the medication as directed on CD 3 and Ron administered the Fertinex™ shots in my thigh for me. I went back to the doctor on CD 12 in early January for the follow-up ultrasound.

The exam revealed that my ovaries had responded well to the prescribed dose of medication. I had follicles on my left ovary at 18½ and 18 mm, and my right ovary had follicles at 21½, 20, and 28 mm. Since everything looked so good with the development of these follicles, my doctor told us we could proceed with the Profasi™ shot. And, since we were already at the office, the nurse could give it to me then. That was OK by us. That meant that Ron wouldn't have to administer it that night. Good thing they reminded us to bring the Profasi™ with us to our appointment.

Once again we were instructed to have intercourse approximately 32-36 hours after the Profasi™ shot was administered. This is the approximate time in which the follicles would release the eggs. So here we go again. I was highly medicated and had a swollen, sore belly, but I was eager to conceive a child. Ron, of course, was always gracious and patient with me.

We had an opportunity to get our minds off waiting for the results by going skiing with our church youth group. We chaperoned a three-day skiing trip with two other couples. Ron and I had tons of fun and were envious of the other parents on the slopes teaching their small children how to ski. We couldn't wait to have the chance to teach our children as much as we could. I couldn't wait to see the sparkle of spirit and adventure that appears in a child's eyes when they have just learned how to do something new.

Cycle # 10 - Summary

CD 3	150 mg Serophene™
CD 4	150 mg Serophene™
CD 5	150 mg Serophene™
CD 6	150 mg Serophene™, 2 amps Fertinex™
CD 7	150 mg Serophene™, 2 amps Fertinex™
CD 8	2 amps Fertinex™
CD 9	2 amps Fertinex™
CD 10	2 amps Fertinex™
CD 11	2 amps Fertinex™, ultrasound
CD 12	10k unit Profasi™

We returned from our ski trip on a Monday and I started cycle # 11 by Wednesday. I was only on CD 25, so I was caught off-guard. Of course, I called the doctor's office to let them know about the onset of my cycle. They had me go to the lab for a blood test to confirm. When the blood test came back negative, she asked me to come in for an ultrasound. She wanted to see what my ovaries looked like. We saw several small follicles on each ovary. The doctor explained that we would have to coast a month to let the ovaries "recover" from cycle # 10. The small follicles were left over from the previous cycle and they needed time to shrink back down before stimulating them again.

I didn't quite understand this and asked her why we just couldn't keep "feeding" the ones that were already there. Time was wasting! The last thing I wanted to do was wait yet another month without treatment. I do not remember her exact reply, but I think the answer was tied to egg quality and maturity. So, disappointed as usual, I went home to wait for this period to end and then an additional month for the "coast" cycle. I was to report back to the doctor when I started my *next period*. I considered the coasting month cycle # 11, even though I wasn't going to ovulate.

There was a small problem with this idea though. Since history proved that I couldn't ovulate on my own, I probably would not start the next period after coasting. And I did not. By late February, CD 30 came and went. I called the doctor's office. They called in a prescription for Provera™ in order to bring the onset of a period. I received the generic, Cycrin™, from the pharmacy. I took 10 mg of Cycrin™ for seven days and waited. No period. I called the doctor's office again and stated that I had forgot to tell them that the Provera™ generic had not worked on me in the past. Therefore, they called in a script for Provera™ again, this time no generic allowed and they doubled the dosage. I took 20 mg of Provera™ for seven days and waited. Finally on CD *50*, I started cycle # 12 in mid-March.

We wasted all that time trying to bring on my next period and, unfortunately, we would have to wait even longer for further treatment. Ron was sent on a business trip to Indonesia that lasted 30 days. There was no sense in seeking treatment if Ron was not available. We had also planned a vacation after his return and knew that it would be very difficult to pursue treatment in the midst of all the traveling. So we were told to call the office when we were ready to begin another treatment cycle.

This time I was OK with the delays. Since my low point a few months prior, I had gained better perspective, as had Ron. After returning from his Indonesia trip, he went to work for a new company that required less travel time. At the same time, I was analyzing my career goals.

I was convinced that I needed to leave my job, but I didn't want to make any rash moves without discussing them with Ron first. So we discussed my feelings, and wanted to see what his thoughts were. I had questioned my career for several reasons. The first reason was that I, of course (type A personality that I am), had this master plan of our life laid out and I structured my career moves around this plan. This plan consisted of having a child in the spring of 1997 and one in the fall of 1999. And now the reality was that this may not happen, either at all or at a time undetermined by me. The result of this master plan was that I stayed in a position that did not require heavy traveling, in order to make it easier to become pregnant. Therefore, I was feeling unchallenged by the job I had been doing for several years.

The second reason was that I had been re-evaluating the direction my life was taking. My soul searching earlier in the year led me to feelings of selflessness and charity. I felt an overwhelming urge to want to do some volunteer work. Work that would allow me to help others. I wanted to give of myself, without being paid for it. However, stepping out from under the corporate umbrella would create uncertainty. It wasn't the uncertainty of finding fulfilling and challenging work, it was the uncertainty of the further cost of fertility treatment and insurance coverage. If I left my job of eight years then, I'd be giving up my insurance benefits and income. With Ron just starting his new position at a new employer, it was a bit risky. And since the risk was greater than the possible rewards at that time, we decided that I couldn't quit right then. But if things went well with his new job, we were going to revisit my ideas in six months.

About a month after Ron and I had our conversation, all of a sudden there was a dramatic change at work. My direct supervisor retired on short notice. I was now the only person that carried the information on how to perform the department's requirements and also knew all of the history. This changed the playing field for me. While the work got more intense, it got much more interesting. And I loved it. I was working quite a bit, even while seeking my medical treatments. But I had even more energy than ever now.

By April 1998, we had been trying to get pregnant for two years. But looking back at the cycles, I really only had twelve cycles, or twelve good chances to conceive by that point. Comparatively, women that ovulate regularly each month would have had twenty-four cycles over the same timeframe.

Up to this point, we had only spent approximately $550 on out-of-pocket costs for treatment. "Treatment" included doctor visits, ultrasounds, medications, blood tests, and home pregnancy kits. The total out-of-pocket costs without medical insurance would have been approximately $3,000. Luckily for us, the injectibles were covered under my company's prescription card. This is what saved us from financial strain. Our out-of-pocket costs were still pretty high over the long haul, but it could have been much worse. The injectibles are a small fortune by themselves. If the injectibles had not been covered on my prescription card, **each** cycle would have cost us approximately $2,300, depending on the number of vials prescribed.

Cycle # 13 - The First IUI

May 1998 – June 1998

In early May, I called the doctor's office to initiate the process for a new treatment cycle. The doctor's office called in a new round of prescriptions. They were all the same as before, nothing new. I started double doses of Provera™ (no generic) for seven days to wait for the onset of cycle # 13.

This was our first attempt again since the January cycle. That cycle had really good follicle response, so the recipe for this cycle was very similar. I was prescribed a triple dose of Clomid™ for five days, followed by 2 amps of Fertinex™ for three days, then report back for an ultrasound. That was when I began giving the subcutaneous shots to myself. Even after our extensive April travel schedule, Ron was still on the road a lot for work. Since he was not at home in the evenings, I administered the shots on my own.

In late May, the ultrasound showed many small follicles measuring at less than 7 mm on the left ovary, and 9 and 9½ mm, on the right. This was a very different response than the January treatment. I had measurements of 18-28 mm over the same timeframe during the last cycle. My doctor told me to take a triple dose of Fertinex™ each of the next three days and come back in for another ultrasound.

I went to the pharmacy to pick up 9 more amps of Fertinex™, and went back to see my doctor three days later. The new scan showed follicles of 14½, 14½, 13½, and 13½ mm on the left ovary and 15½ and 15½ mm on the right. We had progress, but they were not large enough yet for release. Once again, I was sent away to take a triple dose of Fertinex™ for two more days and return for another ultrasound. Off to the pharmacy again. Six more amps of Fertinex™ and two days later I went back in. It was now CD 16 and I had follicles measuring 17, 16, 15, and 12 mm on the left and 19, 17, 15 and 13 mm on the right. She said that we were ready for the Profasi™ injection. From our previous conversations, I thought that the follicles needed to be at least 18-20 mm. So I asked her to explain why we were proceeding with small follicular size. She said that a small amount of the Fertinex™ would remain in my system for another day and would continue to "feed" the follicles making them grow just a bit more. So we proceeded with the administration of the Profasi™ shot. The eggs would release in approximately 32-36 hours.

My doctor added something new to this cycle. She wanted to check the effectiveness of the Profasi™ shot by having me use an ovulation predictor kit (OPK) that evening. The result from this test should verify that the Profasi™ did stimulate an elevated LH hormonal change, and therefore, triggering ovulation. The over-the-counter OPKs detect LH hormone in urine. LH is the hormone that releases an egg from the ovaries.

Dr. Gold also suggested that we try an intrauterine insemination (IUI) on this cycle. The last cycle looked so good, but was not successful with natural intercourse. The IUI is a procedure in which the doctor places the sperm directly to the back of the uterus, bypassing the cervix, cervical fluid, and lower portion of uterus. This means the sperm only have to swim through the fallopian tubes to the ovaries, where the eggs are released. By bypassing everything else, it increases the chances of sperm meeting an egg. And hopefully, fertilization!

We agreed to try an IUI for this cycle. We scheduled the procedure for the following afternoon. Before we left the doctor's office, we were given a sperm collection kit. It included a specimen cup and some paperwork. The instructions made it clear to make sure that we had our names on the specimen cup and sign off on the paperwork <u>before</u> we came back to the office.

I bought my OPK at the hospital pharmacy on my way back to work. There were different brands of kits and most were in the $35-40 range. I chose one that cost $35. After reading through the instructions at home that evening, I determined that the test was simple and easy to use. I just had to urinate on five different sticks for five days in a row and watch for the stick to change colors.

The next morning we got up bright and early. It was our first attempt to collect the semen sample in the morning before work. Once the specimen was collected in our <u>labeled</u> cup, I raced to the doctor office with the cup under my shirt in my bra. I know it seems ridiculous, but it is a great way to keep the fluid warm. The collection cup is about the size of a large shot glass. Once I reached the doctor's office, I handed the cup and the paperwork off to the lab technician. The lab put the specimen through a process called a "sperm swim-up" or "sperm washing."

The first step in a sperm swim-up separates the sperm from the seminal fluid that they swim in. To accomplish this, they are placed in a nutrient medium and then in a centrifuge. Once the fluid has separated, it is taken from the top and discarded. The remaining sperm are mixed again with the nutrient medium for a second ride in the centrifuge. This process is meant to separate the weaker sperm from the stronger sperm. The remaining sperm are then drawn into a syringe with an attached catheter (long plastic tube).

Ron and I referred to this procedure as the shower and shave procedure. We thought it was a great analogy. The sperm were getting "cleaned up" for their adventurous quest to find an egg to fertilize.

The IUI process is usually painless. Sometimes people feel a bit of a cramp, but it does not require anesthesia. To do an IUI, the doctor inserts the speculum to open the vagina. The doctor then feeds the catheter with the semen specimen through the cervix and into the back of the uterus. The syringe is then emptied, releasing the sperm into the uterus.

Sometimes the IUI process is reserved for those clients that exhibit difficulty with sperm or semen quality. Even though Ron's previous semen analysis came back with good motility (the strength to swim up to the eggs), the IUI would increase our chances by 10%. Even that small of a percentage was worth it to us. The IUI was like placing the sperm at the door. All they had to do was go through the door and go in.

Unfortunately, my doctor was traveling that day, so her partnering doctor performed my IUI. This procedure should have gone very smoothly, but my body did not cooperate. We discovered that I have a tipped uterus and a funky curve through the cervix. I had never had an IUI before, so we were both in uncharted territory.

After the first few attempts to insert the catheter without success, the technicians had to take the sperm solution back to the lab. Apparently, the sperm solution in the catheter cannot stay out of the incubator away from heat for very long. The doctor kept attempting to get the catheter through, and now of course, it wasn't as painless as it should have been. The nurse ended up having to push on my lower abdomen to get my uterus tipped down. Remember I already had abdominal swelling and tenderness from stimulating my ovaries, and now they were pusing down on that very area, really hard. I just held my breath and looked at the ceiling. It only took a few more attempts before he got the catheter positioned properly. And boy, could I feel it. They retrieved the sperm solution from the lab and inserted it through the catheter. Then the nurse asked me to lie there for 20 minutes. There is no evidence that lying down increases the success rate, but they always suggest that it doesn't hurt.

When my time was up, I got dressed and exited the exam room. The doctor additionally advised that we should continue to have intercourse starting the next evening. It would increase our chances of conception.

I paid $250 for the IUI as I left the doctor office. I had already researched our medical coverage and knew that neither of our insurance companies would cover the procedure.

We followed the doctor's orders to continue having intercourse over the next few days. As painful as it may have been for me, I was willing to do just about anything for positive results. We had gone so far up to this point and we added the IUI, how could this cycle NOT work! My OPK results were also perfect. It reflected the color changes on the correct days, which confirmed the detection of the hCG hormone. This in fact verified that the Profasi™ did induce ovulation. . My stick had a slight pink tint to it and when it detected a higher level of hormone, it became a darker pink.

Everything looked really good for this cycle. But unfortunately twelve days later, I started cycle # 14.

What is wrong with me? The results were quite a let down. What could have gone wrong now? We had even added the IUI and the OPK this time. I was sure that this cycle was a "sure thing."

I called in to report the onset of my cycle. My doctor asked me to come in for an ultrasound to check the status of the remaining follicles. This time I had many small follicles on both ovaries and she said that we needed to coast again for one month to clear out the old follicles. I had to wait at least thirty days, then call the office if I did NOT start a period.

I was really bummed… The thoughts of a family for Ron and me keep getting further and further away.

Cycle # 13 - Summary

CD 3	150 mg Clomid™
CD 4	150 mg Clomid™
CD 5	150 mg Clomid™
CD 6	150 mg Clomid™
CD 7	150 mg Clomid™
CD 8	2 amps Fertinex™
CD 9	2 amps Fertinex™
CD 10	2 amps Fertinex™, ultrasound
CD 11	3 amps Fertinex™
CD 12	3 amps Fertinex™
CD 13	3 amps Fertinex™, ultrasound
CD 14	3 amps Fertinex™
CD 15	3 amps Fertinex™
CD 16	10k unit Profasi™, ultrasound
CD 17	IUI

Cycle # 14 – A Time to Reflect

June 1998 – July 1998

Cycle # 14 was during June and July 1998. Since I had to "coast" a month before any new treatment could begin, I spent most of my time trying to reconcile myself with so many feelings of despair. I still often felt anger, sadness, jealousy, pity, and anxiousness, even *after* I gained perspective in the spring. I don't know what happened to me. It is so hard to stay emotionally high and energetic, when each cycle seemed to age me by ten years. I am sure the colossal hormonal changes are a bit to blame. It's like such a crazy roller-coaster, up and down, up and then down again. Sometimes I had to focus on just getting through the day. It takes an unbelievable amount of energy and stamina to continue a positive outlook. It's exhausting.

I admit now that before my infertility trials, I was hungrily trying to achieve my goal list. I worked a lot of hours (and loved it), traveled (and loved it), and worked to prepare our new house for a family. With my checklist in hand, I was eager to check off the next "goal" I had to achieve. Setting goals is not necessarily a bad trait to have, but I had such a sense of urgency and impatience. There was no room for time delays. I thought that is what life was all about; setting goals, reaching them, and setting more. When I was not pregnant within the first six months of trying, it was like a punch in the gut. What do you mean I'm not pregnant? I had a mission to complete. I had originally planned on our first child to be born sometime in the spring of 1997 (since we started trying in August 1996) and the second to be born sometime in the fall of 1999. Not for any reason at all other than it fit into my "life plan." I thought that I'd like to have two children about 2½ years apart. I never shared that detail with Ron. I'm sure when he thought he might like to have a family someday, his thoughts didn't go to strategizing the month in which they would be born and how far apart they'd be.

As the negative results continued endlessly, I became more frustrated and angry. Why couldn't I control this part of my life? Other people could and with great ease (it seemed). I was so angry that I did not have a body that worked like clockwork. Feelings of jealously, bitterness, anger and sadness still overwhelmed me at times. And before I could stop, these feelings consumed my every thought. Then one day, a light came on. If I continued being jealous and angry all of the time, it would change the essence of who I was. Did I want that to happen? No! I knew that I did not want to be perceived as a mean, bitter, angry, nasty person. Which meant that I couldn't be a mean, bitter, angry, nasty person on the inside. All of these emotions were negatively affecting my energy, and sucking the life out of me. I needed to find a way to better control these feelings, but I didn't know how to do it.

I started to travel quite a bit by myself with my new responsibilities at work. This seemed to take my mind off the stress of fertility treatment, at least temporarily. I knew it would be there when I returned.

During this time of travel away from normal day-to-day operations, I observed. No matter where I was, in the airport, dining alone, or walking in a new city, I just loved to observe people. All kinds of people: old, young, male, female, Americans, foreigners, business-dressed, and vacationers. As I watched people around me, I thought about how different each and every one of us are. And even though we are all different, we are uniquely tied together to each other through relationships. We nurture these relationships, and they are the backbone of the society that we create and share. A society that cares about others, and one that depends on these interrelationships to exist. What happens to us when we sometimes let this important nurturing in our lives get away from us? It isolates us from what is most important, each other. Of course, we all have responsibilities that have to get done, and goals we want to achieve. Sometimes this can cause us to lose sight. (Have I lost sight?) Unfortunately, it usually takes a shattering event to reshape the priority levels that we have. If we each had to reduce our needs and desires to just a few items, what becomes *most* important in our lives? I realized what is most important to me. In my world, it is nurturing relationships with loved ones - spending time with them, sharing moments, celebrating life; and also important to me is the work that each of us can do to help build a better society. I appreciate and treasure all of these moments, because that is what is important to me.

I was slowly learning that I could not be in control of everything. A *very* difficult task for me. What if we weren't meant to have children naturally? I needed to loosen the grip that I had on my "list". I also would need to figure out a way to accept the cards that I had been dealt, and move on! No feeling sorry for myself anymore. I had been given a body that needed some extra special attention, and I needed to now learn, at 27 years old, how to make it work. That meant changing old habits and establishing new routines. Then one day it just hit me...

PROCLAMATION: I need to take care of my body inside and out. This is the body that I was given to live in. I have to depend on me to live my life. Be at peace with myself. And develop a way to find acceptance with myself. Then live my fullest LIFE.

Amidst all of my frustration, I remember a moment in which I recognized all of the good things that I had in my life, my husband, my job, our home, and our health. These are very fortunate things! Others are not as lucky. I think we easily take these for granted while trying to achieve more. It seems like after this occurred to me, then everything else became much clearer. What's really important in my life shot to the top of my priority list. I needed to stop feeling sorry for myself and realize that I have it much better off than many others do, beginning with a wonderfully compassionate husband, who has been my lifeline of support.

During this time of reflection, I also realized that children are absolute miracles sent from the heavens, and life itself is beautiful and should be lived pursuing your greatest dreams and desires. Some people waste a great deal of their lives being completely miserable for various reasons. Our time on this planet is so short, we have little time to be miserable. For the first time, I started to become very comfortable in my skin.

I realized that I've taken much for granted in my life; people, relationships, security, shelter, food. I'm ashamed that I really never thought about it. But we are all surrounded by so much every day, it is easy to take it all for granted. I hope to be more grateful. And to celebrate simple things such as a sunny day, the birds singing and the excitement of children playing on a playground.

It was at this time that I decided to share the past two years of frustration with my mom. I had not previously told her everything, for two reasons. First, I dreamed of the day I would get to surprise her with a pregnancy announcement and secondly it is sometimes difficult to always be asked how treatment is going, when it does not go well. But I thought it was probably unfair to keep her in the dark about the treatments, and she must be wondering what was going on by now. So I spilled my guts.

She didn't seem as surprised as I thought she would be. Like I said before, I think a mother's intuition led her to believe that something was wrong. I explained that I had begun to tell Jen on our trip last summer about some of the difficulties we were having, but made my sister promise not to say anything to her. Since then, we had new treatment plans and were still trying.

My mom told me that her sister, my aunt, had difficulties conceiving thirty years ago. They think her problems were probably thyroid gland-related, but back then they didn't have anything to help determine that. Maybe this was something I should have checked out, my mom said. I explained what our treatment plan was focusing on, and I explained what my doctor was doing to help me ovulate, which is the first thing that has to happen in order to achieve a pregnancy. I told her that so far I had been treated with medication and had some favorable responses to it. We just had to keep trying until we got the "recipe" of medication correct. I assured her that I was going to be OK. She was very sympathetic to our situation and said she was there for us if we needed help in any way.

Cycle # 15

July 1998 – August 1998

I waited until CD 30 came and went, then called the doctor's office to report in. They called in a prescription for Provera™, one 10 mg pill for seven days. My instructions were to report to the office when my period started. Very quickly, three days after starting Provera™, I started cycle # 15.

Dr. Gold prescribed a new round of medications and said we were going to try something different this time, no Clomid™. I was to follow a new Fertinex™ "recipe" for each day: 3 amps, 3 amps, 2½ amps, 2½ amps, 2 amps, 2 amps, 1½ amps, then return for an ultrasound.

The ultrasound showed one follicle on the left ovary at 10 mm and 11½ and 9½ mm on the right ovary. Now I understood that those were not big enough. My instructions were to take 2½ amps of Fertinex™ that night, then 2 amps per day for two more days. The next ultrasound showed the left ovary had follicles of 13 and 12 mm and the right had 13 and 11½ mm. Once again, new instructions. Take 3 amps of Fertinex™ for the next four days and come back for an ultrasound.

Now mind you, I was running to the pharmacy for additional vials of Fertinex™ and insulin needles in-between going to the doctor appointments, during lunch breaks, and work hours. I wanted to make sure my time at work was made up for, in all fairness to my employer. But, I was always working late anyway because our company was working on a divestiture (opposite from a merger) at the time. This required a lot of extra work on everyone's part. I wanted my manager to know that I could be counted on to pull my weight. Up to this point, there were only three co-workers that were aware of my treatments, and my boss was not one of them. These dear friends were very compassionate during each treatment cycle and were there to listen when I needed to unload my frustrations.

After thirteen continuous days of injectibles, we went back in for yet another ultrasound. This time we saw follicles of 18 and 14 mm on the left and 17½ and 17 mm on the right. Dr. Gold said to go ahead and administer the Profasi™ that evening and follow the standard intercourse instructions. She wanted us to have intercourse that night, the next night, and the third night. She also told me to pick up another ovulation predictor kit. This once again would guide us to the most optimum time to for intercourse after ovulation has occurred.

We talked about whether it made sense to do another IUI or not. I cannot remember why we decided that time NOT to do the procedure, other than the previous difficulty we faced getting the catheter placed correctly and the out-of-pocket cost to us. But I do not think that cost was a major factor, because the IUI was relatively inexpensive at $250 compared to the costs of all the ultrasounds, blood tests, and medications.

If I didn't start a period in two weeks, I was to have blood drawn for a pregnancy test. Again.

Cycle # 15 - Summary

CD 4	3 amps Fertinex™
CD 5	3 amps Fertinex™
CD 6	2½ amps Fertinex™
CD 7	2½ amps Fertinex™
CD 8	2 amps Fertinex™
CD 9	2 amps Fertinex™
CD 10	1½ amps Fertinex™, ultrasound
CD 11	2½ amps Fertinex™
CD 12	2 amps Fertinex™
CD 13	2 amps Fertinex™, ultrasound
CD 14	3 amps Fertinex™, ultrasound
CD 15	3 amps Fertinex™
CD 16	3 amps Fertinex™
CD 17	3 amps Fertinex™, ultrasound
CD 18	10k unit Profasi™

Cycle # 16 – Introduction of Lupron™

August 1998 – September 1998

Ron and I had been working like crazy since April, and I talked him into taking some time to unwind. I searched for a private vacation refuge that we might like. We decided upon the small East Coast town of Cape May, New Jersey on the Atlantic Ocean. To spice it up a little bit, we rented a red Mustang convertible and drove the ten-hour trip to New Jersey. I know this seems like a twenty-something crisis, but I had the overwhelming urge to step out of our structured, predictable life schedules.

We were two days into our trip and were very surprised with the onset of my period. I suppose we shouldn't have been surprised, because it did come on CD 30, <u>AND</u> we were on vacation (so it was a sure thing). But I was convinced that I was pregnant. I had even packed an HPT kit to test around cycle days 30-32. Unfortunately, it made for the remaining days at the beach uncomfortable for me. It figures!

This was the onset of cycle # 16. I called the doctor's office while still on vacation to report in. They said they were going to call in a prescription for something brand new, and I needed to start taking this medication daily on CD 21. It was called Lupron™, and it was an injectible just like Fertinex™. After beginning the Lupron™ on CD 21, I was to wait for the onset of my period, then call the doctor's office.

When we returned from vacation in late August, I picked up the new prescription at the pharmacy. The Lupron™ came as a solution in a vial, no need to mix dry power with saline. However, it needed to be refrigerated at all times. The syringes were smaller than the type that administered Fertinex™; they were the size of a standard insulin syringe.

Lupron™ is a GnRH analog[12]. The purpose of a GnRH analog is to neutralize the FsH and LH hormones coming from the pituitary gland. This allows the FsH (Fertinex™) and LH (Profasi™) to be directly fed to the follicles through the injections without any possible unwanted mid-cycle surge of LH coming from the pituitary gland. My doctor noted that some start regular menses after just taking Lupron™. Yay! After one year and eight cycles with our fertility doctor, we were on to something new. Maybe this was my ticket to success - Lupron™.

I had started taking Lupron™ on CD 21 and after 18 days without the onset of a period, I called the doctor. She suggested that I come in for an ultrasound so that we could take a look at what might be going on. The ultrasound revealed that there were many follicles on my ovaries at multiple sizes. She said she thought that what might very likely be the case was that these follicles were "leftovers" that had been getting some food before I took Lupron™. With the withdraw of FsH and LH, they should shrink back down. I had my blood drawn that day to test what is called

---

[12]   Analog – the purpose of an analog is to oppose the hormone.

an estradiol, or E2, level. This was just the beginning of many, many times that I would have my estradiol level checked.

There are three different types of estrogen produced in the female body. Estriol (E3) is produced by the placenta and is important only in pregnancy. Estradiol (E2) is the most potent and main estrogen in reproductive-age women. Estradiol is almost exclusively produced from the developing follicles of the ovary and can be used as a marker of follicular growth during drug therapy for infertility. And estrone (E1) is the major by-product of estradiol as it is cleared from circulation. Estrone is the most common estrogen produced after menopause and is used in some hormone replacement therapy (HRT).

My E2 came back that day at 692 which, at the time, meant nothing to me. So I asked what kind of number we were looking for. She said that a rule of thumb to follow is that each matured follicle that is approximately 20 mm in size should produce an E2 level of 200 pg/l (picograms per liter). This number can be all over the board in a polycystic woman. She could have many small follicles emitting small amounts of E2 totaling more than 200, or one large follicle that is emitting high amounts of E2. Since we were at the beginning of this cycle, when follicles should be less than 5 mm, we were looking for the number to be around 50.

She explained that, as the FsH and LH were being restricted through Lupron™, the follicles should shrink back down, therefore lowering the estrogen output and E2 level. And since my E2 was 692, she could tell that I did indeed have some estrogen-producing follicles. We waited a week to do another ultrasound.

Now, all this time I was still taking Lupron™ - twenty-seven days worth. The next ultrasound, seven days later, was virtually the same, except now I clearly had one follicle taking over. It was distinctly larger than the others. Because of this one follicle, we didn't get a blood test. The size of this follicle showed that the E2 would be high. She wanted me to stay on Lupron™, and I needed to come back in one week to monitor the (hopefully) shrinking follicle.

I was now on the thirty-fourth straight day of Lupron™ injections. I went in for another ultrasound and found out that the one large follicle was now *huge*. So we named that one the "FsH hog." It was monstrous and was kicking out a boat-load of estrogen, so the E2 level would not decline. I asked if the follicle was going to produce an egg and if it was, why couldn't it be released, fertilized, and see if we hit the jackpot. She stated that the egg quality was probably poor, if there was even an egg inside at all[13]. Okay, I thought, so maybe that wasn't such a good idea, but I learned something new.

Then Dr. Gold said in a matter of fact tone, "Do you want to drain it?"[14]

---

[13] According to <u>PCOS: The Hidden Epidemic</u>, "We know that the oocyte (egg) that is ovulated past day 14 is much more likely to be defective. Delayed ovulation occurs often in PCOS, virtually every time the cycle length is over 30 days. Not all eggs subjected to intra-follicular aging are defective, but statistically the risk is higher." Pg 50.

[14] This is not something that you have to do on every circumstance. The alternative was to take Provera™ again for 5 days, wait for a menstrual cycle then check again to see if the follicle shrunk.

Drain it? Just like that. Drain the FsH hog and force it back down to a normal size. I asked, "How?"

"We'll put a needle at the end of the ultrasound wand, go in, puncture it, and drain it."

I thought it sounded easy enough. So I said, "Sure, go ahead."

She said, "Oh no, not today. We have to have more time. How about tomorrow?"

And without any hesitation, I said "That will be fine," even though I knew I was swamped at work and couldn't afford to be away. It was pretty stressful to have to keep leaving the office for each appointment, not because of the missed time, but because I wanted to be discreet about my ordeal. Ultimately any time from the office during the day would be made up by staying late into the evening. We made the appointment for late the next day, and I made arrangements for my co-worker and friend, Denise, to drop me off and Ron to pick me up.

Draining a Follicle

October 1998

When I got to the RE's office, I was surprised that we went into what I'll call a "surgical" room. Hmmm. I thought we would be in the regular exam room with the regular stirrups and the ultrasound machine. But this room was larger. It had a really big bed and the bed had leg pads at the end to rest your legs in. The ultrasound machine was the only piece that was the same. Oh, except for the fact that there was a needle fixed to the end of the ultrasound wand. This needle had a flexible plastic tube attached that was hooked up to a motor. Pretty neat stuff. Talk about interesting! I am amazed at the advancement of medical procedures. In just a matter of minutes, a doctor can insert a tool into the vagina, view the ovarian follicle, prick it with a needle and drain the contents into a tube. The procedure sounded pretty simple. It seemed to me that my doctor and her staff treated this procedure as fairly routine.

So, the description of the procedure is simple. Insert wand, view the ultrasound monitor, locate the follicle (or sometimes called a "cyst"), puncture it, turn on the motor, suck out the contents (or "drain it"), turn off the motor, and withdraw wand. Sounds easy enough. Well, that's not how mine went, of course.

I got up on the table, laid back, and rested my legs in the leg rests. They fired up the ultrasound machine and wheeled the machine with the motor right up next to it. The speculum was inserted first, and then the ultrasound wand was inserted with the needle attached to the head. Dr. Gold explained everything as she went along, and all was well.

As she put pressure on the follicle to puncture it, we saw on the monitor that it kept rolling around. And then something hit me in just the right location and sent excruciating shots of pain down my right leg - kind of like when you pinch the sciatic nerve in your lower back. I was squeezing Ron and Sandy's (my nurse) hands so tight that they had to switch sides of the bed. My eyes instantly filled with tears, and Ron kept his eyes focused on my face. I must have had a horrified look on my face, because he continued to reassure me that it would be okay, we were almost done. After what seemed like an eternity, Dr. Gold decided to withdraw and try again after a break. Clearly, I was very uncomfortable. She said that it shouldn't have been that painful. I kept saying that there was a pain shooting down my leg.

After about 5 minutes, everyone came back in to try again. I readjusted myself and got prepared. This time I looked at the ceiling when she went in and in about 30 seconds, I heard the motor turn on, then off, then she was withdrawing the wand.

She said, "That's it!"

"You're done, that's it?" I questioned. I didn't feel anything except for the pressure from the ultrasound wand.

"That is how it usually goes, but the follicle kept moving out of the way when I tried to puncture it the first time."

I thought about it a little after we were done, and I think that the fact that I was lying on my back and had a little bit of pressure near the base of my back near my sciatic nerve may have created the sharp pain down my leg. By all means, this ended up to be a piece of cake.

The lab technician examined the fluid that was extracted from the follicle and determined that there was no egg within the follicle.

So the "hog" was drained, and I went back in for blood work four days later. My E2 was at 71, which was much lower than the 692, but we were looking for it to be under 50. An E2 of 50 or lower gives a pretty good indication that there aren't any stray follicles still developing.

In the meantime, we consulted with Dr. Gold for the next course of treatment. We decided to do another ovulation induction[15] cycle with an IUI. Therefore, we were given prescriptions for 40 amps of Fertinex™, one 10 k amp of Profasi™, one 5 k amp of Profasi™, and a refill for my Lupron™. Now, up to this point I had been taking Lupron™ injections for 39 days, and my last period was 59 days ago. And I still needed to continue taking Lupron™ throughout the next cycle.

Eight days after draining the follicle, my E2 level came in at 56. That was our green light to start the next treatment cycle.

I was particularly irritated during this cycle because it had been 64 days since the beginning of my last period. I know that the "hog" follicle was to blame, but this "waiting game" is agonizing. I've never experienced such anxiousness in all my life. All in all, we were 2½ years into this now, with not ONE positive pregnancy result!

---

[15] Ovulation Induction (controlled ovulation stimulation) – use medication to stimulate several follicles to develop on the ovaries.

Cycle # 17 – My Mistake

October – November 1998

My new recipe of medication called for 3 amps of Fertinex™ and one shot of Lupron™ each day for 12 days, followed up by an ultrasound. An unbelievable thing happened this time!! It was picture perfect. We had never seen such beautiful follicles. The left ovary had one at 21 mm and two at 20 mm. The right ovary had three at 20 mm. OUTSTANDING! We finally did it. This is it. Perfect little eggs inside those follicles just waiting to be released and fertilized.

I had a blood test after my ultrasound that day and my E2 was sky-high at 3944. I was reminded again that the general rule of thumb is that each 20 mm follicle can emit approximately 200 pg/l of estradiol. I had six large follicles and many other smaller ones. The six larger ones would have emitted approximately 1200 pg/l, but my E2 was much higher than that. So the nurses told me that I was "On Fire," which was their way of saying I was full of estrogen. I did discover a bit of truth to that phrase though. When my estrogen was high, I felt invincible. I had tons of energy, my thought processes were quick, precise, and clear. I didn't notice the "estrogen highs" at first as much as I started to notice the "progesterone lows." I will explain this soon.

There are possible health risks associated when the E2 comes back at such high levels. One is ovarian hyperstimulation syndrome. Therefore, Dr. Gold told me that I needed to "coast" a day. Coasting just meant that I did not need to take any injections that night, and I had to go back the next day for another E2 blood test. Coasting allows time for the smaller, less mature follicles to shrink back down, therefore lowering the E2. When the E2 has reached an acceptable level, the Profasi™ (hCG) is administered to release the matured follicles.

My next appointment fell on a Saturday morning. My regular blood lab at the doctor's office complex was closed, so we went to the blood lab at the hospital. Ron and I were sitting in the reception area of the hospital, waiting for the blood lab technicians to report to their station. There were two other woman sitting there with us. I presumed that one was a patient of Dr. Gold's, because I had just seen her leave Dr. Gold's office at the same time we did. While we were waiting for the hospital receptionist to arrive, I sat and wondered what each of my waiting room partners had been through - their pain and their struggles. Sometimes conversations creep into these moments and can surprise you. Why is it that we find comfort in knowing that there are other people out there going through the same painful process? I think we find comfort in community, thus reducing our fear of isolation. In other words, sometimes we find incredible strength, perseverance, and determination in ourselves when we see that others have weathered the same storm.

The blood lab technician showed up and called all three of us back at the same time. It was a quiet walk down the winding set of hallways that led us to the lab. We each stood lined up in the order we walked in and waited while the lab tech grabbed the paperwork and called the first name. It wasn't mine. It was the woman who came in first. As I stood with the other woman and waited, I said, "I suppose we are all checking for the same thing? Hormone levels?" Well, you would have thought the Hoover Dam gave way. We each spent the next ten minutes telling an abbreviated version of "our story," all while getting our blood draws. When we were finished, we wished each other to be the next success case. We each had different degrees of infertility, but struggled privately just the same.

My blood draw results determined the E2 level had fallen to 3287. That is a 657 point drop in one day. We were given the okay to administer the Profasi™ shot that evening at 11:00 p.m. That would make the timing for the IUI at 9:00 a.m. Monday morning.

As in the past, we collected the sperm sample in the early hours of Monday morning. I raced it to the lab by 7:30 a.m. and then proceeded to work. I left work around 8:45 a.m. in order to get to my appointment on time. This was old hat to me now, so I was pretty calm and relaxed. Dr. Gold performed the IUI, and I had to lay on the table for about 20 minutes with my knees up. She still had some difficulty getting the catheter in, but not nearly as bad as the first time. I had them put a small pillow under my butt, because lying on the hospital bed flat on my back for 20 minutes usually hurt my lower back.

Sandy came in to tell me that I could go, and reminded me to take the booster Profasi™ shot that evening.

"What booster shot?" I asked.

She asked me if the doctor prescribed an extra 5k vial of Profasi™ for me.

I said, "Yes. I thought I was to mix the 10k and the 5k together and administer at the same time. I did not know that I was to keep the 5k for a separate booster shot." She looked at me kind of funny and then left the room for a bit. When she returned she told me that I needed to call the doctor immediately if I had any difficulties over the next few days. She explained that I may get sick, because of the extra Profasi™ that I had taken. They went over the symptoms to look for. At the time, I really didn't think anything of it.

Before I left the office, my doctor gave me a prescription for progesterone suppositories. I was to insert one tablet vaginally twice a day. A progesterone supplement is prescribed especially when Lupron™ has been used in the cycle. Lupron™ (GnRH analog) has the advantage of blocking an unwanted LH surge from the pituitary gland and ovulation, but also suppresses the production of progesterone (P4) that is naturally triggered by the LH. This P4 type of progesterone is needed to thicken the uterine lining to prepare for the fertilized egg to implant.

Remember that without the production of LH and FsH, the ovaries will not produce follicles. That, in turn, decreases estrogen and progesterone which are needed to sustain a pregnancy; this is why supplemental progesterone is given.

There is also something called progestin that I referred to in "The First Attempt." The brand names are Provera™ and Cycrin™. Progestin is a synthetic agent that mimics the action of progesterone. It is more commonly used to make you start a period. The medication itself does not cause your menstrual cycle to begin, but it is the withdrawal from the medication, or when you stop taking it, that induces a period.

I remember going back to work that day and thinking about the cycle. It was the most perfect cycle so far. How could it not take? The follicular response and growth was perfect, and everything looked really good. I was so eager for the results, but would have to hold in the excitement for two weeks. During those 14 long days, we just hoped and prayed that it was our turn for a miracle, because that is exactly what children are!

Wow, I learned something new again. The progesterone suppositories were easy to put in, but extremely messy after a few hours. It left a white, cakey substance in my underpants. My suggestion would be to wear panty liners after the administration of the suppositories. Otherwise, you'll be changing your underpants a lot.

This was my first time on the progesterone supplement. Dr. Gold explained that it is the progesterone's job to thicken the uterine lining for implantation of the fertilized egg and to maintain the pregnancy in the early stages. If you are deficient in progesterone, it is likely that even a fertilized egg may not implant in the lining, or may implant for a short time before being shed with the next menstrual cycle.

I was extremely uncomfortable and sluggish, and my abdomen was tender and painful. My IUI was on Monday, and by Friday I was nauseous and getting through work was a chore. By Friday night, I couldn't eat and tried a little chicken broth but immediately threw that up. I even tried a glass of water and later threw that up. I didn't get much sleep that night; getting comfortable was impossible. I am a belly sleeper and that was not an option. The swelling was miserable. I wondered how pregnant woman slept at night, they couldn't be nearly as uncomfortable as I was. By Saturday morning I couldn't stand it any longer, and I called my doctor's office.

I explained to the receptionist how sick I was, and that I was having a difficult time with the pain. Dr. Gold got on the phone and told me to go right to the hospital. She was pre-admitting me and would meet me at the hospital later. I was a little caught-off-guard about being admitted. I thought that see would have me go to her office and maybe prescribe a painkiller, but I wasn't expecting a hospital visit.

My illness was definitely going to affect my plans that I had for that Saturday. In addition to working a full time corporate job, I am also a freelance photographer. Predominately, my business consists of photographing weddings and major events, and on that particular Saturday I had an all-day karate tournament booked to shoot. I promptly called my client to explain what was happening to me, and unfortunately had to cancel the coverage. That was the first time I EVER had to cancel my services. I was horrified. But I knew that I could not physically complete the shoot that day. He was understanding and wished me well. All I kept thinking about later on was "Thank God the event wasn't a wedding," because I was *really* sick, and it is nearly impossible to find a replacement photographer on the day of a wedding.

Ron drove me and my vomit bucket to the emergency room. When I arrived at the desk, I told them my name and they escorted me right to Admitting. They processed the paperwork quickly and assigned me a room immediately. I was wheeled upstairs with my bucket on my lap. Within 20 minutes of arriving at the hospital I was in a bed, had an IV inserted, and the Morphine administered. Then they added an anti-nausea medication to the IV drip. I was finally feeling calmed and relaxed. The meds in the IV didn't take away the pain and swelling in my abdomen, but it made me comfortable.

I found out that I had a good case of ovarian hyperstimulation syndrome or OHSS - sudden ovarian enlargement. The symptoms are abdominal pain; abdominal distension (which means "enlargement"); gastrointestinal symptoms including nausea, vomiting and diarrhea; severe ovarian enlargement; and weight gain. I had every single one of those symptoms. In severe OHSS there is fluid accumulation in the pelvic and abdominal cavities. Occasionally this extends to the area around the lungs called the pleural cavity. Depending on the degree of severity, it may be necessary to drain the fluid from these areas to relieve the intense pain. The procedure to remove the fluid from the abdominal cavity is called paracentesis. The greatest concern with this syndrome is that the loss of fluid from the blood vessels creates a concentration of blood cells and increases the possibility of blood clot formation. There is a slight chance of death with OHSS. One of the major concerns with ovulation induction is the potential for OHSS.

In the days following my IUI, my belly had been so sensitive to the touch that I wore very baggy clothes all week. When I took my clothes off at the hospital, Ron gasped at how swollen my belly was. He couldn't believe how quickly it had set in. He felt really bad. He said that even though he saw me every day, he hadn't seen me with my clothes off and was shocked at how swollen my belly was when I undressed for the hospital gown. I suppose that I looked four to five months pregnant, because I had gained approximately 5-7 pounds since the IUI on Monday.

My doctor came in that evening and explained to me what was happening and what I was feeling. She explained that the ovaries are located in the pelvic area, just about between your pelvic bones. In the case of OHSS, they become so enlarged that they come up out of the pelvic area and, because of the limited amount of room in the abdominal cavity and the extra fluid that has been produced, put pressure on the diaphragm. This was so very painful and was the cause of my shortness of breath. The pressure on the diaphragm made me feel like I couldn't breathe. I could only take short shallow breaths; it felt as if someone was sitting on my chest.

She told me about the procedure that they could do to relieve some of the pressure in the abdomen. This was the paracentesis. They could drain the fluid from the peritoneal cavity (abdomen) through a tube, relieving some of the pressure. I agreed to try it.

After we talked about what takes place during a paracentesis, she and the nurse gathered the supplies that they needed to perform the procedure. They came back with a syringe filled with some kind of numbing agent, a large needle with a catheter tube attached, iodine swabs, cotton balls, and a bucket on the floor. She poked around my belly with her finger, found a good spot, numbed the surface of the skin with the shot, waited a few minutes for that to set in, then stuck the needle with the syringe into my abdomen, and started to suck on the other end with her mouth, like a siphon. The fluid started to come out! She pointed the plastic tube over the bedside, into the bucket on the floor, and we watched as it started to fill up. I couldn't believe that I had a catheter stuck in my belly and fluid was running freely out into a bucket on the floor! She asked me how much fluid I thought would drain? How much fluid did I think was in there? I didn't have the foggiest idea. She and the nurse were commenting about other patients that have had 2 liters drained at once. Two liters! That's like a plastic pop bottle full of fluid sitting in someone's abdominal cavity! That was amazing to me.

I don't remember how much fluid we drained, and I didn't happen to keep my journal back then, but it filled up the bucket and had to be emptied for more. After the fluid stopped coming out, she felt around for any other "pockets" of fluid and then pulled out the needle. Ahhh. I felt so much better. I could breathe again, and deep breaths were possible. It felt like so much weight had been lifted off of my chest.

I ended up getting drained again on Sunday, as the swelling seemed to reach its peak. Then I began to urinate on my own again, and the swelling started to reverse. The nurses recorded all fluid in and out of my body the whole time I was there, so that my kidney function could be monitored. And they checked my body weight a couple times a day. At the peak of the swelling, I had gained seventeen pounds to 157 pounds from my normal carrying weight of 140. This was approximately over a 4-day period of time. Every time I got on the scale, I couldn't believe how quickly and how much fluid weight I had gained. Once again, I didn't know that was possible.

Once the process begins to reverse itself, meaning the kidneys kick in and start to discard the fluids naturally, the highest risks are over. That was when they gave the approval to be released from the hospital. There was still some pain and swelling in my abdomen, but Dr. Gold prescribed some medication for pain management.

I was released on Monday afternoon and was told to stay home from work the remainder of the week to rest. Dr. Gold asked me to come in for a blood test on Tuesday morning for an early pregnancy test. It had only been one week since the IUI, but she wanted to check it anyway. The beta level came back on Tuesday at 9. And at the time, I had NO idea what that meant. They told me that it meant that I was slightly pregnant and I had to continue taking the progesterone suppositories and rest, rest, rest. I later discovered that according to the lab they use, beta results of 0-5 are negative. So this didn't mean negative. It meant very close to negative.

This was the best result that I had <u>EVER</u> gotten. So, I was asked to come back again on Friday for another test.

The test on Friday was not as encouraging. It was 6 and not looking good. The number was declining for one, and it was extremely low.

One more beta test on Monday concluded it was over. It was less than 5. Not Pregnant.

This was such a tragedy for me. It was such a beautiful and perfect cycle. We had come further than ever before on this cycle, so I should have been pleased. But all I could think about was my misunderstanding on the Profasi™. The doctor told me that the extra medication is not what caused the loss of this cycle, the extra medication caused the OHSS. But I still blamed myself. Everything looked so good, and I was so ready! I would endure OHSS a hundred times over just for a positive pregnancy test.

It was a very sad time at our house and our extended families. Everyone was concerned about my health and the OHSS that took over my body. Then to add to it, the negative pregnancy results. However, it was a time that Ron and I bound even closer together. I drew on him for his physical strength to help me with everyday tasks, and I needed his comfort when I had to cry and vent my frustrations. If he was being affected by all of this, he didn't wear it on his sleeve. I knew that he was sad and discouraged, but only because we talked about it in private. I, on the other hand, physically looked like I had been hit by a truck. And the mention of the word "baby" in a conversation would throw me in to a tither. I felt like I was losing my way...

Even though I knew my life was good and even though I knew I had a great marriage, I still got very caught up in the sadness of each loss. I don't know how to explain the emotional sacrifice that I put out for each cycle. It's like I wanted to only have positive thoughts so that it would generate positive results. And when those results come back as negative, you get slammed.

I was ready to just throw in the towel and say forget it. I had had it with everything: the fertility treatment, the job, the frustration, the costs, the hurt, the anger, the sadness. I was so tired, so finished. I was so worn out...

As soon as my period started, I intently grieved this unborn child. The beta level number in the blood test was an indication to me that *something* had happened. Maybe an egg and sperm *had* fertilized and created an embryo? Maybe that embryo had implanted in the endometrial lining and was now shedding right before my very eyes. Maybe nothing happened at all, but we would never know. I was so heartbroken, so sad...

I dragged myself through the next few weeks. Wake up, get out of bed, drive to work, cry on the way, get to work, try not to cry all day, leave work, cry on the way home, eat dinner, and try not to consume my evening with all that had happened. In the midst of all of this, at work we reached the conclusion of the large project that we had been working so hard on. It was at least a bit of a relief to have that finished and complete. We were just heading into the holiday season and things would be a little quieter at the office.

When I spoke to my doctor at the time of the final blood test, she had asked us what we would like to do regarding future treatment. She suggested that we wait awhile and heal our hearts, then after we'd had time to think about everything, give her a call back with our decision. She said that we were sooooo close last time. The beta level was actually positive for a few days, which meant that I *could* become pregnant. That was not questionable anymore.

Ron and I each had been going through our grieving process. I don't think any of us know just how much time we need individually to heal until we are faced with such difficult moments. I know that I spent my time crying and dreaming about our lost child. This seemed to help me heal my heart for this baby and, from this process, I gained the strength to continue on. It was a feeling of renewal and cleansing. It was as if I needed to devote that time to those feelings of loss and defeat. And when I woke up one day and the hurt finally stopped hurting so much, I knew it was time to move on. I was much more at peace. The phrase, "time heals all wounds," does have a bit of truth to it, even though when we live through the anguish, it seems impossible healing will ever come.

When Ron and I discussed moving on, he asked me if I was ready to handle yet another round of emotional sacrifice. I said that I didn't know what I could handle until it stared at me in the face. We would just have to put one foot in front of the other and trudge through. I was bound and determined to find out a way to make this work. After all, we had found out that I *could* get pregnant. So, we agreed to call Dr. Gold and begin treatment again.

Cycle # 17 – Summary	
CD 1	3 amps Fertinex™, Lupron™
CD 2	3 amps Fertinex™, Lupron™
CD 3	3 amps Fertinex™, Lupron™
CD 4	3 amps Fertinex™, Lupron™
CD 5	3 amps Fertinex™, Lupron™
CD 6	3 amps Fertinex™, Lupron™
CD 7	3 amps Fertinex™, Lupron™
CD 8	3 amps Fertinex™, Lupron™
CD 9	3 amps Fertinex™, Lupron™
CD 10	3 amps Fertinex™, Lupron™
CD 11	3 amps Fertinex™, Lupron™
CD 12	3 amps Fertinex™, Lupron™, ultrasound
CD 13	15k units Profasi™
CD 15	IUI
CD 20-22	OHSS – Hospital stay
CD 23	9 - Beta level (pregnancy test)
CD 26	6 - Beta level (pregnancy test)
CD 29	<5 - Beta level (pregnancy test)

Cycle # 18

November 1998 – January 1999

I called my doctor to tell her what we had decided. We discussed a treatment schedule and she asked me to begin taking the Lupron™ injections, but it had to be at least 21 days after my last period. I only had to wait a couple more days to get to CD 21. She wanted me to come back after two weeks of Lupron™ injections for an ultrasound.

After two weeks of Lupron™, my ultrasound in early December showed that my ovaries were not swollen any longer, and they had several small follicles, but no "hogs." This was good news and the green light to go forward. This would be Cycle # 18. She prescribed 30 amps of Fertinex™, and a 10k amp of Profasi™. We knew that I needed Lupron™ to neutralize my FsH and LH hormones and 3 amps of Fertinex™ a day for ten to twelve days to get my ovaries to respond properly. Since the last cycle unveiled a successful recipe that we knew worked well, I was excited to try again. We must be so close! During the last cycle I had 3 amps of Fertinex™ and Lupron™ for 12 days and BINGO, perfect follicular development.

However, I never asked but I think my hyperstimulation stayed on Dr. Gold's mind. She backed way off on the recipe for this cycle. The cycle recipe was .10ml Lupron™/each day plus the following amps of Fertinex™: 3, 3, 3, 2½, 2½, 2½, 2, 2, 2½,

December 30th was CD 10 and my ultrasound showed follicles on the left ovary at 12, 12 and 9 mm, and the right ovary had 12 and 10 mm. The blood test showed my E2 level at 595. This cycle was looking good. We were seeing good follicle growth and the hormone levels seemed appropriate for the size of the follicles. Instructions were to continue Fertinex™ for three days at 2½ amps, 2, and 2 then return for another ultrasound. Ultrasound #2 was on a Saturday, and it showed follicle measurements on the left at 18, 17, and 11½ mm and on the right 15, 13½, and 16½ mm. I was told to stop taking Fertinex™ and come back on Monday so that they could check my E2 level and perform another ultrasound. This would allow me to coast a couple days to prevent OHSS again. Ultrasound #3 on Monday, displayed follicles on the left ovary at 21, 19, and 16½ mm and the right at 18 mm, and my E2 level was at 827. Dr. Gold gave instructions to administer the Profasi™ injection late that evening, at approximately 11:00 p.m., in order to have good timing for an IUI on Wednesday morning at 9:00 a.m.

Off I went to the doctor's office on Wednesday morning at 7:00 a.m. with the sperm sample nestled inside my bra again. We had to keep those little soldiers warm. (I always wondered what I'd say if I were pulled over by a police officer, with such delicate cargo on board, but that never happened). They got dropped off to the lab safely, and I headed to work.

I was running on pure adrenaline then. I was swamped at work and working late hours. We were closing out our fiscal year and it required about two weeks of late evenings. There are only a certain number of days available to complete the financial information for publication and disclosure.

On Wednesday, I headed to the doctor's office for my 9:00 a.m. IUI appointment, greeted the staff when I arrived, and welcomed the sight of the little vial that was going to make me a Mommy. The sperm had had their shower already that morning, weeding out the weakest and leaving the strongest swimmers to attack my eggs.

This time around, I did NOT take 15k of Profasi™. She only prescribed 10k anyway, so we never had the risk. After verifying my name on the vial that contained the sperm solution, my doctor inserted the catheter. As Sandy pressed down on my lower abdomen to flatten out the curve in the cervix, Dr. Gold loaded up the syringe with the sperm solution, and delivered them to the back of the uterus. The procedure went smoothly this time. I had to rest on the bed for 20 minutes with my knees up, and I started daydreaming about the baby we were creating. I wondered how it was ever possible for people to conceive that weren't even trying. This was unfathomable to me. There are **so many** factors, (egg, sperm, fertilization, and implantation) that have to be lined up just right for a pregnancy to happen. It is so miraculous!

So there I was, in the middle of the absolute busiest time of the year for me at work, and I had already had a full day by 9:30 a.m. Once again, we were trying to create a miracle. It can be a humbling experience.

Fourteen days later, unfortunate results. The beta level was 1.

I started my period on January 22nd and mourned the loss of this cycle. Even though we got the pregnancy result two days prior, the start of my menstrual cycle finalized it. I just cried and stared at the blood leaving my body. Although we'll never know if there was ever an embryo, maybe there was and it just didn't adhere to the uterine lining. I was mourned the loss of another child that could have been.

By this time, when we told others of our infertility; we were told that we just needed to relax. They would say, "Amy should just quit her job and reduce the stress level in her life and she'll get pregnant. She works too much anyway." The funny thing is that I've never really been one to feel really "stressed out". I know what it is like to be very busy at times, but not really emotionally stressed from it all. I enjoy the work I do.

I did receive a copy of an article from a friend on how stress affects fertility. When anyone would see anything on infertility, they would send it to me. This article referred to the Goddess of Infertility, a psychiatrist that counsels infertile couples through their sadness and despair, and they usually end up getting pregnant. Was that the cause of our problem, stress? I just couldn't buy in to the thought that ours was stress-induced infertility. I had never menstruated regularly in the past. The tests conducted thus far have revealed that my hormones and ovaries do not produce consistent follicular growth, which is vital in order to produce a healthy egg. I was sure that our infertility was caused by physiological irregularities. I wished so much that I was a normal female, with normal cycles. I would welcome the monthly period, if it meant it would bring me that much closer to having a child of our own.

Before any other treatment could begin, we had to sit out one whole cycle again in order to clean out the leftover follicles from the previous treatment. Yet another agonizing waiting game.

We once again started to discuss the remaining options with our doctor. We talked about the possible reasons that the forms of treatment we had tried were not working and what may have been preventing pregnancy results. But these questions are nearly impossible to answer from the doctor's point of view because if they knew, they'd treat it. This time the discussion included in-vitro fertilization (IVF).

What did IVF provide that the other treatments did not? Was this our only chance, our last resort? We did not even know if IVF would work for us, and like all other treatments, it did not come with a guarantee. What were the increased chances statistically? We had so many questions: the cost, any insurance coverage, health risks, concerns over multiples, etc.

After lengthy discussions together, Ron and I decided that we were going to try IVF for the next cycle. Maybe this would get us one step closer. At this time, we also began to think about the possibility and complexities of adoption. We had compared the cost of IVF to the cost of an adoption (approximately $10,000), and we figured we could try two IVF cycles for the roughly the same cost. I still wanted to try to exhaust every attempt for me to become pregnant. The cost at our doctor's facility for the IVF procedure was going to be $4,200, which did NOT include the cost of the pre-surgery fertility medications. The breakdown of the $4200 was:

- $2500 IVF package at the hospital
- $720 retrieval of eggs
- $450 anesthesia
- $360 embryo transfer
- $170 ultrasound guide

The fees for the IVF procedure would be a direct out-of-pocket cost to Ron and me. We knew at that point that neither of our insurance companies provided IVF coverage (and there are not many that do). However, the injections were still covered under my employer's prescription card.

I had done as much research as I could on the Internet regarding IVF procedures at other fertility facilities in the country, and it seemed that we lucked out. Our local area was one of the lowest-cost areas that performed this procedure. I saw costs that went as high as $10,000 for one cycle, not including injections. Some centers even had "package deals" that did include all injections for a much higher price tag.

Cycle # 18 – Summary

CD 1	3 amps Fertinex™, Lupron™
CD 2	3 amps Fertinex™, Lupron™
CD 3	3 amps Fertinex™, Lupron™
CD 4	2½ amps Fertinex™, Lupron™
CD 5	2½ amps Fertinex™, Lupron™
CD 6	2½ amps Fertinex™, Lupron™
CD 7	2 amps Fertinex™, Lupron™
CD 8	2 amps Fertinex™, Lupron™
CD 9	2½ amps Fertinex™, Lupron™, ultrasound
CD 10	2½ amps Fertinex™, Lupron™
CD 11	2½ amps Fertinex™, Lupron™
CD 12	2 amps Fertinex™, Lupron™,
CD 13	2 amps Fertinex™, Lupron™, ultrasound
CD 14	coast
CD 15	10k unit Profasi™, ultrasound
CD 17	IUI

Cycle # 19 – InVitro Fertilization

February – May 1999

We proceeded with our plans for in-vitro fertilization this cycle. We had not achieved a pregnancy during the most recent four cycle attempts that used ovulation induction coupled with an IUI, so we wanted to move on.

In-vitro fertilization refers to a process in which eggs are retrieved from an ovary and placed in a petri dish with the sperm. The contents of the petri dish are monitored by the lab technicians for fertilization and the results are documented. When and if an embryo does develop, it is placed back in the uterus.

The procedure sounds very easy; however, that is the very simplified version of what needs to take place. There are many factors involved with each step and with each step comes the possibility for complications. The process begins with inducing follicular development via injectible hormones, then monitoring the hormonal levels with blood tests and monitoring ovary response by ultrasound. When the follicles are large enough, the eggs are surgically removed. There is the possibility that the number of eggs retrieved or the quality of those eggs may not be acceptable to proceed. Once the eggs are in the dish, the sperm is added.

After the sperm and eggs are joined in the petri dish, fertilization must occur. If fertilization does not occur, the process is over. If fertilization does occur, the fertilized eggs may or may not fully develop into viable embryos. In the meantime, medication must also be taken by the patient to prepare the uterine lining to receive any viable embryos. If viable embryos develop, they are transferred into the uterus. The embryo then needs to "hatch and attach" itself to the uterine lining. Hatching is an easier term for referring to the process in which enzymes break down the wall of proteins around the egg called the zona pellucida (ZP).[16] And attaching refers to when the egg attaches to the uterine lining. As you can see, IVF is a highly technical procedure, with many steps to achieve a successful pregnancy. It is highly emotional as well, with many ups and downs. Each step brings new concerns, but it gave me a renewed sense of hope.

Before our attempt at IVF, we never even knew about the "hatch and attach" process. This was another new piece of information that we learned. We just could not believe yet one more piece of the puzzle that had to be completed in order to conceive a child. How do the cells know what to do? And how do they know when to hatch? It is simply miraculous that children are born at all.

At that time, we went to each of our family members to discuss our decision with them. We wanted to explain the IVF procedure and all the steps involved. Many were concerned for my health because of the OHSS reaction that I had had five months prior. I explained that it was very unlikely that something like that would happen again. If I did hyperstimulate again during this procedure, the

---

[16]   PCOS: The Hidden Epidemic – "The ZP prevents attachment of the embryo to the wall of the fallopian tube as it travels down to the uterus. Once in the uterus, the ZP dissolves and the embryo "hatches"." Pg . 209

embryo transfer would probably be delayed until I returned to normal. Hesitantly, everyone wished us well and said they would pray for us.

To launch this cycle, we began Lupron™ in late February 1999. It was to be followed up by an ultrasound and blood work in nine days to check on the follicles and my E2 level.

Well, what do you know? I had another "hog." There was a huge follicle that was lingering around, and it was throwing out a large amount of estrogen. My e2 level was 774.

Here we go again. Nothing seems to ever be easy for me. Maybe I'm just being tested to see what kind of endurance I have. Sometimes I believe that you honestly never know how strong you are, or what you are capable of, until you are pushed to your limits.

The doctor and I quickly decided that we would schedule to drain the follicle the next day. I was better prepared this time and understood what needed to happen, and everything went as planned. There were no mishaps with back pain like the last time.

After the follicle was successfully drained, I began taking an antibiotic. This is a standard precaution for the IVF procedure. It is taken to protect the body from any type of infection that could inhibit the egg retrieval process. Unfortunately, I had a reaction to this antibiotic, and my chest and belly area broke out in a rash. By the time the rash developed, I was almost done taking the pills. So we just let it go and it eventually went away when the antibiotic wore off.

I went back in on Monday three days after the follicle was drained for a blood test and my E2 was 124.2, a considerable decrease from 774, but not low enough. I was told to get another blood test the following Monday, one week later.

In the meantime, I was to stand up for my best friend who was getting married in Las Vegas that weekend. The travel wasn't going to be an issue on timing, because we were waiting for the E2 level to drop down below 50. However, I was still on Lupron™ all this time and it needed to be refrigerated. So we needed to get creative.

Ron and I found a small, insulated lunch box that would at least keep the contents cold. If we packed the Lupron™ in ice in a Ziploc bag, it would stay cold during the flight until we reached our hotel room. Once we reached our hotel room, we used the ice bucket to store the ice that kept the lunch box cold. Our arrangement worked out rather nicely. I continued taking the Lupron™ injections without any interruptions.

The Monday that we returned from Las Vegas, I went in for my blood test. It was 10 days after the follicle was drained and my E2 was 48. Perfect! Hooray!

So, the very next day I went in for an ultrasound to double-check the ovaries before we proceeded. I had follicles that were measuring in at less than 4 mm and my endometrial lining was at 3 mm. This was good news, of course. I was told to go ahead and start my injections of Fertinex™ and to also continue the Lupron™. The goal was to try and achieve a good number of quality eggs to retrieve without overdoing it. If we overdid it, it was likely that I could have hyperstimulated again, and then retrieval and transfer would have become much more difficult; so difficult that the embryo transfer could have been canceled or delayed.

This time my recipe called for .10 ml of Lupron™ and 3 amps of Fertinex™ for eleven days, then come back in for an ultrasound to monitor the growth. I could tell something was definitely happening by eight days into the injections because my belly was really tender, bloated, and achy.

We went in for the ultrasound and blood test on Saturday, March 27th. My E2 level was astronomical at 7084. However, it was in line with the number of follicles appearing in the ovaries. They were chock full of maturing eggs, and the endometrial lining was measuring in at 12 mm, which meant that it was nice and thick with nutrients to support the growth of an embryo. I asked what size the lining needed to be. And she explained that she wanted it to be at least 12 mm for this cycle. I asked what was normal. She said under normal circumstances they like to see it thicken to approximately 9-12 mm depending on the patient. She instructed us to administer the hCG injection that night. By taking the 10k Profasi™ at precisely 11:00 p.m. that evening, the eggs would be ready for retrieval at 7:00 a.m. Monday morning, March 29th. I also had to take one antibiotic pill on Sunday to prevent reproductive tract infections, just as a precaution.

I had asked if I could return to work after the retrieval procedure, but my doctor said that I would be slightly sedated for the procedure and could not drive the remainder of the day. Therefore, I had made arrangements to take Monday and the day that the transfer would take place as vacation days. However, the transfer day is not known until the fertilization and growth progress of each embryo is complete.

The night before the surgery, we reviewed the paperwork that had to be filled out and turned in to the office in the morning. One sheet was the standard sperm collection document, and the other packet was about the IVF procedure. The document asked questions regarding our intentions for the retrieved eggs/embryos after the procedures. Questions that we had never thought of, for example were: if there were extra embryos produced, and they were frozen, which of us would be granted rights to those embryos (in the case of a divorce); where would they be kept and for how long; and who was responsible for paying the storage fee. We were both required to read, fill out, and sign these forms. These were legal precautions that had never even crossed our minds before. There were also moral and ethical questions like, what to do with the possible unused extra embryos? Are they destroyed, donated to science, or donated to another couple? These are tough things to face up to and decide on.

Monday morning we crawled out of bed around 5:00 a.m., showered, and got dressed. I put on my most comfortable pair of sweats and sweatshirt. Then, of course, we had to collect Ron's little soldiers, for they too would have to be showered and cleaned up for their performance in the petri dish date later that day. After the collection took place, I packed the cup in their warm riding place and off we went.

I'll never forget the drive into the doctor's that day; it was a bright, beautiful spring day. It felt like a perfect, fresh new day to become parents. The journey to the office was quiet. We didn't really discuss much. We had a huge anticipation of success; both of us were excited to believe that this would be the end of treatments and the beginning of parenthood; the end of frustration, and the beginning of sheer joy. Here's to the end of the piling medical bills and to the beginning of scraped knees and elbows! Only one word seemed to describe our state that morning: hopeful.

The procedure that I would undergo was first practiced in England. In the summer of 1978, the first "test-tube" female baby was born. Now twenty-one years later, Ron and I were finding that our future was at the mercy of this amazing procedure. Our prior knowledge up until then, had really only been what the media, via television, radio, newspapers, and magazines, had reported on the subject. We have all seen and heard of super-multiple births and surrogate pregnancies through media coverage. However, after our experience thus far, I wished that large sets of multiple births wouldn't become a media event. Most likely, behind each of these stories is a couple that probably struggled for years before their prayers were answered, and that is the story that is not usually told. I now have a much better understanding of the trials and decisions that these families have had to make.

Well, when we finally arrived at the office, it was pretty early, but my doctor and her staff were in their scrubs waiting for us. We handed off our release forms and the sperm. They, of course, would be getting prepped for their debut later today. I kissed Ron good-bye and was led back to the surgical room. He would stay in the waiting room while the surgery was taking place. He brought along his laptop that day so that he could work while the hours went by.

The surgical team consisted of my doctor, two nurses, two lab technicians, and an anesthesiologist. Amazingly, I was very relaxed, very peaceful. The anesthesiologist started an IV in my right arm and said that I would start to feel a bit drowsy. I remember asking if I would be "knocked out" completely or just groggy. He said that it would be like a light sleep, but I wouldn't be awake. That's the last thing that I remember.

As I awoke, I looked around as if I had only been asleep a few minutes. There were only two people in the room, the anesthesiologist and one of the two nurses, Donna. I asked if they were already done. She said, "Yes, it went very well." Then Dr. Gold came in with Ron right behind her. She said that they had retrieved thirty-eight eggs. My eyeballs popped! Thirty-eight! Holy cow! I was astounded! "Everything went very well," she said, "the hard part is over, now we will be watching them closely as the sperm solution is added."

The doctor handed me a couple of ultrasound pictures that she took of the follicles on the ovaries prior to beginning the surgery. There were so many. I couldn't believe it. They are pictured in Figure A.

Each dark black
round form
indicates a follicle
on the ovary that
contains an egg.

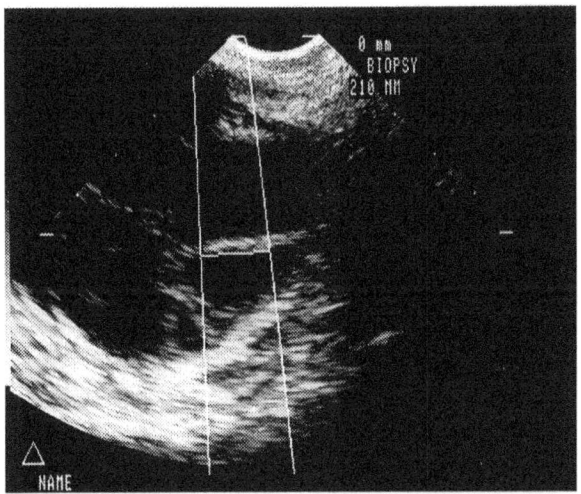

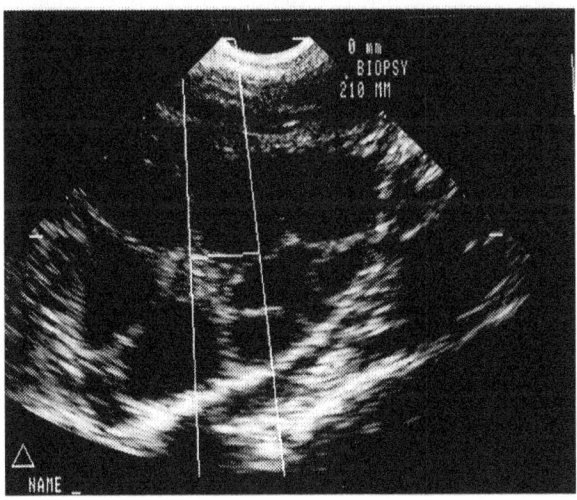

Figure A – Follicles Cycle 19

The lab technicians came in and explained what the next few steps would entail. They would be putting the sperm solution in with the eggs later on that day. The next step was to hope for fertilization and development of what is known as a zygote (two-cell stage embryo). After the sperm penetrates the egg and fertilization occurs, the oocyte (egg) develops a hard shell around it (zona pollucida), begins dividing (also called cleaving). A fertilized egg quickly divides into a two-cell embryo, then from 2 to 4-cell, then from 4 to 8-cell and so on. Once the embryos reach the eight to ten-cell stage, they are then transferred back into the uterus. The lab technician, Taylor, said she would be calling me each day with progress reports on the developments in the petri dishes. At that point we did not know which day the embryo transfer would take place. It is all based on the success in the petri dishes. Hopefully, we would be back later on in the week for the transfer. Everyone had their fingers crossed!

Because of the anesthesia, I was instructed not to drive for the remainder of the day. I didn't seem to be in too much pain, but definitely felt achy. My doctor said not to be alarmed if I bled a little bit, and she suggested wearing a panty liner.

I slept most of the way home. I do recall, though, through my groggy haze, that a policeman pulled Ron over on the expressway for going a little bit too fast. Luckily, Ron explained what we had just endured and that he wanted to get me home quickly. The officer was very understanding and let us go on our way.

When we reached our home around 10:00 a.m., I couldn't wait to get into my own bed and sleep. I would be returning to work the next day, so I wanted to get as much rest as possible. Ron made sure that I had everything that I needed, and then he headed into the office. He said that he would call me later to check up on me.

"I'm doing okay," I said when he called, "just sleeping a lot." He asked if I needed him to come home to help me with anything. I told him no and that I'd probably still be in bed when he came home that evening.

I did get up and go in to work on Tuesday. I didn't feel bad, just a little battered and tender in the abdominal area. But that was expected. I was at my desk on Tuesday when I received the call from Taylor. She said, "thirty-two of your eggs fertilized, six did not." She also said that that was a very good percentage rate of fertilization, 32 out of 38 is 84%. Dr. Gold said that the *average* percentage of fertilization in their lab is 85-100%.

When I returned to work on Tuesday, my three co-worker friends, Denise, Rose and Jane, asked how my surgery went. I went on to explain to them what stage of the process we were in at that very moment. After I told them that our biological contents were in petri dishes at the lab and could be creating our child as I spoke, they each commented at how truly amazing it was that medical advancement could get us this far.

I was also at work on Wednesday when Taylor called me. She said that of the thirty-two blastocycsts[17], thirty-one continued to split and form multi-cells, and one went flat. I asked what "going flat" meant, and she said it showed no

---

[17]   Taylor referred to an embryo as a "blast", so I looked the term up. Blastocyst refers
        to the stage of embryo development just prior to implantation.

further signs of development. Everything looked very good, and they scheduled the embryo transfer for Thursday morning.

I made arrangements to take Thursday off work, and luckily Friday was Good Friday and our offices were closed in observance of the holiday. Normal protocol calls for resting off of your feet for a few days after an embryo transfer to give them every chance to adhere to the endometrial lining. If you strain or try to lift heavy objects, you have the risk of losing the cycle. They didn't have to tell me twice. I had nothing but rest planned for the days following the transfer.

Ron drove me to the doctor's office on Thursday morning for the insertion of the embryos. We were led back to the same procedure room as when they extracted the eggs. This room happened to be directly connected to the lab by a small sliding glass window; this makes transporting the embryos to the procedure room much quicker and more convenient. When we arrived in our room, we had an opportunity to look at our little embryos on a television monitor. The lab records the progress of the embryos in each petri dish on videotape. It was pretty amazing to the both us that each of these little developing cells was our DNA, our baby, our child. I just sat in awe.

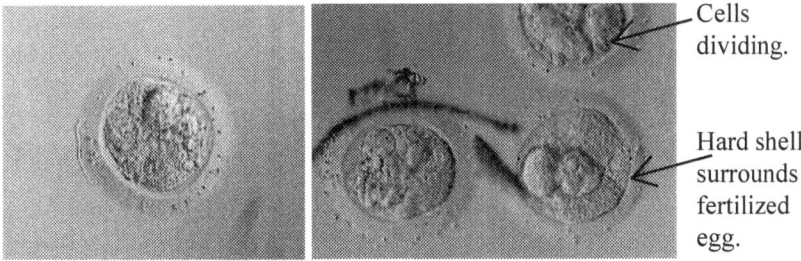

Cells dividing.

Hard shell surrounds fertilized egg.

Figure B –Embryos of Amy and Ron Hansen

At that time, Ron and I discussed with my doctor how many embryos should be implanted. We, of course, had enough for an entire kindergarten class, but the goal here was for a healthy pregnancy and a healthy baby. The doctor suggested that we insert three of the strongest-developing embryos, and the rest of them would be frozen. We agreed. I don't remember what the exact numbers were, but I seem to remember each embryo having about a 33% chance of survival. I could live with that. One in three and we were inserting three. This meant, statistically, that we were there!

This procedure was almost the same as an intrauterine insemination. The speculum was inserted into the vagina and opened, and a catheter was inserted past the cervix and into the back of the uterus. Once again, the nurse had to help push down on my abdomen to allow the catheter to get through the cervix. This time, it was terribly swollen from the stimulation and retrieval process and it hurt like hell. But... I had gotten that far, I wasn't going to turn back.

Once the catheter was through, they checked its position in the uterus with the ultrasound unit. They did this by taking the ultrasound wand and pressing it externally on my abdomen. And yes, it hurt as much as when the nurse had to press down earlier with her hands. The catheter location looked good and the strongest three embryos were drawn up from the petri dish into a syringe by the lab technicians and were transferred from the lab to my room. Then Dr. Gold connected the syringe to the catheter and released the embryos into my uterus. They kept the ultrasound wand on my abdomen the entire time in order to monitor the insertion of the embryos into the uterus. I could see on the monitor where the fluid with the embryos released from the catheter. The only noticeable difference between my previous IUI's and this transfer was the use of the ultrasound machine to monitor the insertion.

That was it! I felt different. I was finally going to be pregnant with our child… I could not go to church on Easter Sunday. I lay very still all weekend.

Ron and I chanted for the next week or so "hatch and attach," "hatch and attach." It didn't have to be all three, just one would be fine. We would find out in two weeks.

The pregnancy test was on April 15, 1999. I had my blood drawn in the morning before work, as usual. And I received the call from my doctor at work. She said, "Amy, this is Dr. Gold, I am so sorry… The test came back negative." How incredibly devastating! How could I do anything else, but burst out crying. I had to get up and shut my office door so that no one could hear me or see me. I couldn't believe it. I was so sure this was going to be it. What was it going to take for us to get a successful cycle? It was just so unfair. All of that preparation, the surgery, the anguish of the procedures, and not to mention the costs involved. We could have paid for a few years of college by now. Why was this happening to us?

My doctor was very kind and sympathetic on the call. We talked for just a few more moments while I choked back my tears. She asked me to report in with her when my period started.

I called Ron at work shortly after to tell him the results; and he was always very good at comforting me. He always knew exactly what to say. It had to be disappointing for him too, but he knew I was very upset. He suggested that I go home and get some rest. So, I went home early that day from work. I just wanted to be at home to grieve. I didn't want to talk to anyone and didn't want any questions. I wasn't even prepared to talk about this to my friends that knew about the procedure.

I was so very sad…

I just cried and cried. Was I doing something wrong? Maybe I strained myself too much after the surgery? I could not think of anything that I could have done to have overdone it. Why didn't the embryos attach to my lining? Was there something wrong with my uterus? I was so full of doubt, anguish, and sadness. A part of the deep sadness I felt was because I knew that the embryos were alive when they were transferred into my uterus and evidently they did not adhere to the lining. My heart ached for the three little embryos that were implanted because, to me, they were a living part of me. They were the closest we had ever been to having a child. They were, in my eyes, our children…

I was also very angry at the "waste" of the money. Apparently, this should not inhibit my feelings, but the fact was that we were not made out of money, and it was becoming an issue. We were both hard-working, professional individuals, but this could not go on forever. We didn't have the liberty of bottomless pockets. Thank goodness we were frugal savers. Our earlier years of saving had been funding most of our procedures.

Now it was time to just sit and wait. Wait for the dreaded end to the cycle: my period. The doctor said that it should start at any time. And it did. Later that same day, I started spotting. By the next morning, I definitely knew it was all over. It was hard enough to accept the pregnancy test results, but when the tissue and blood actually left my body, I mourned all over again. It made everything final.

I called in to report the onset of my cycle to the doctor. She asked what we thought we might want to do from here. Her suggestion was to wait awhile to heal emotionally from this cycle, and then attempt a frozen embryo transfer (FET). We still had 27 embryos in the freezer at the lab. I only learned later that we were very fortunate with the number of eggs that were harvested, and that the fertilization percentage was fairly high. That gave us an opportunity to transfer more embryos without having to go through the injections and the full IVF retrieval process again. Sometimes women that undergo the IVF procedure only have a few eggs to harvest, therefore greatly decreasing the odds of a successful pregnancy.

Ron and I discussed what our next step should be. Since I had to wait 30 days anyway to cycle out once before we proceeded with any further treatment, we just decided to use that time to heal emotionally and get prepared for our first FET attempt.

During the 30-day waiting period, we tried to come to grips with what we had just been through. It is such an emotional ride. When you think you have finally come to grips with the results and are ready to move on, someone asks you how it went. Then the feelings of loss come rushing back all over again.

On a positive note, Ron and I concluded that the IVF procedure did at least do one thing for us. It proved that his sperm and my eggs are compatible and WILL fertilize. It never crossed my mind that that could be an issue, but for some couples it is. That was one piece of the puzzle that we didn't know, because we always did an IUI. During an IUI, the sperm are placed in the uterus with the intention of them swimming up to an egg and fertilizing it. There was no way to confirm that his sperm and my eggs ever fertilized in the previous cycles. Unfortunately, this was a pretty expensive way to find out that piece of the puzzle.

Cycle # 19 – Summary

CD 1	3 amps Fertinex™, Lupron™
CD 2	3 amps Fertinex™, Lupron™
CD 3	3 amps Fertinex™, Lupron™
CD 4	3 amps Fertinex™, Lupron™
CD 5	3 amps Fertinex™, Lupron™
CD 6	3 amps Fertinex™, Lupron™
CD 7	3 amps Fertinex™, Lupron™
CD 8	3 amps Fertinex™, Lupron™
CD 9	3 amps Fertinex™, Lupron™
CD 10	3 amps Fertinex™, Lupron™
CD 11	3 amps Fertinex™, Lupron™
CD 12	10k unit Profasi™, ultrasound
CD 14	Egg retrieval surgery
CD 17	Embryo Transfer

Cycle # 20 – Frozen Embryo Transfer

May – June 1999

As we began to gear up for our first FET, Ron and I discussed the possibility of applying for short-term disability coverage through my employer for the recovery period after the FET. After our first IVF attempt, I went back to work immediately. The way I looked at the situation was that I had such an investment in the retrieval of eggs earlier in the year, the least I could do was give the FET everything I had. If I took two weeks off work after the procedure, I could lie down with my feet elevated. This is the critical period of time, when an embryo implants in the uterus. The doctors always say that the less physical activity, the better. I had enough years of service with my employer to qualify for disability coverage, and my doctor said she would definitely approve a leave for medical reasons. The only thing left that I needed was approval from my immediate supervisor. That was the tough part for me. He had <u>no idea</u> of what had been going on all of these years. I had to come clean and explain what we were going through. It wasn't out of embarrassment or humility as to why I never told him, it was because I never wanted to appear "less capable", or "weaker" than my male counterparts. I wanted a level playing field for any promotions.

I knew that this would be difficult for me, because there was a BIG part of me that did not want my work performance to be affected by personal issues, and I didn't want him to see me being emotional. I hated the fact that I cried very easily, especially when it came to discussions about having a baby! I looked at this situation from his point of view and felt bad that I would be leaving during such a busy time for the company and that he only had a couple weeks notice.

I asked him for a moment of his time about three weeks before the scheduled FET. I began by explaining to him that Ron and I had been trying to have children for just over three years, and we had many procedures performed without success. I explained that we had decided to continue on to the next level of treatment. I explained what we had recently gone through in April with the IVF, how that led us to the FET procedure, and the estimated time of return from this treatment. My supervisor has a family himself, and I think he was sympathetic, but a bit surprised. He was very understanding and said that whatever the doctor recommended was fine with him. He said he would approve any disability documents that were needed. He wished us good luck as I left his office.

I proceeded with the paperwork to file for short-term disability coverage. My doctor and my supervisor signed off on them. I was now approved for four weeks of leave starting on the date of my FET procedure.

The preparation for our first FET was yet another learning experience. As I explained earlier, I had to wait 30 days after my last period ended, before any new treatment could begin. When CD 30 came and went, I reported in with my RE. She ordered a blood test to examine my E2 level. This would give an indication as to the hormonal level being generated by the ovaries. My E2 was 66 on CD 33. Pretty low for me, when you look at my history, but she wanted it to be under that magical 50 number. So I went back on CD 37 and it was 63. Then back once again on CD 41 and it was 35. Bingo! I was ready to go.

This time the "recipe" was completely new. It called for 1 estrace (2 mg) pill for seven days, then 3 estrace (2 mg) pills for three days, then back down to 1 estrace (2 mg) pill for five days with 2 cc progesterone oil injections starting on CD 11. This was a new medication regime for me. So, of course, I was well-equipped with questions. Like, why was I taking estrogen pills that are also prescribed to women that were post-menopausal or had had a hysterectomy? I thought that was pretty strange. The doctor went on to explain that we were using the Estrace to trick my body into thinking that I was getting ready to ovulate and the Progesterone to get the uterine lining prepared for a pregnancy.

Basically, to prepare for a frozen embryo transfer, the body needs to "think" that an egg has been released from the ovary, that it has been fertilized, and that it's on its way to the uterus to implant itself in the lining. This is accomplished with the administration of the hormone medications. These medications will help prepare the uterus for pregnancy. Embryos will not survive if they are placed in an unprepared uterus. The estrogen pills raise the estrogen level, simulating what happens just before ovulation. High estrogen levels generate an LH surge, releasing the eggs and progesterone is the hormone that is generated after the LH surge and aids in thickening the uterine lining for successful implantation. If there is a lack of progesterone produced, the uterus may not be prepared to support a pregnancy and the fertilized egg may not implant.

The progesterone that was prescribed this time was in oil form, not suppositories. It came in a vial, just like the other injectible drugs and did not have to be mixed with saline. However, it was a very thick liquid, almost like pancake syrup. We had to administer 2 cc of this oil AND it had to be intra-muscular (in the buttocks), just like the Profasi™ shot. That's where Ron came in. He administered the Progesterone shots for me and, boy, did they take *forever*. It was like pushing the pancake syrup through a pin head. I, of course, had to stand still while he was giving the shot, and I even timed it. It took approximately 2½ minutes from the time he poked the needle in until he pulled it out. It didn't hurt very much, but if he tried to push the liquid in too fast, it would burn a little.

Throughout the new FET treatment process, I did learn something new. Remember when I mentioned the "estrogen highs" and the "progesterone lows" in Cycle # 17? Well in my opinion, estrogen is a wonder hormone and progesterone is not as kind. I soon discovered that I had great concentration and worked very efficiently while on the estrogen patches. I could do many tasks at one time with perfect coordination. It was fantastic. I was a machine. I loved it. But then... I would lose the ground I gained when I was on high concentrations of progesterone. I always felt groggy and dragging. I could read the same document ten times and not retain any information. It was terribly frustrating. I asked Dr. Gold if I was imagining my change of concentration levels. She said that my description of my variable moods were pretty accurate to the effects of each hormone.

On June 2, after nine days of Estrace, I went in for the first ultrasound. She checked the endometrial lining thickness and it measured 9 mm. She said everything looked good and we could proceed with the plans for the FET the following week. The lining would continue to get thicker over the next six days until the scheduled FET.

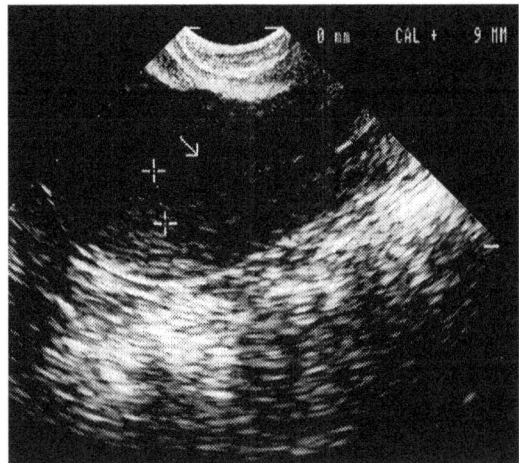

Figure C – Endometrium Lining 9 mm

Our FET was set for Tuesday, June 8, 1999 and my appointment was at 1:00 p.m. I worked frantically until 12:30 p.m. that day to finalize everything before my leave of absence. I was prescribed a Valium pill by my doctor and instructed to take it one hour prior to the procedure time. Because there is no anesthesia administered for this procedure, the Valium was prescribed for relaxation. I had the pill with me that day at work and took it around 12:00 p.m. The doctor recommended that I did NOT drive after taking a Valium, so I made arrangements for my friend, Rose, to drive me to my doctor's office. Ron would meet me there and drive me home.

After we were shown to our room, Dr. Gold came in to explain what the lab had experienced with our frozen embryos. In a previous discussion, we agreed to have four embryos inserted this time, but they ended up having to thaw ten. Here is what happened. The embryos were frozen in small groups, so that when they thaw for an FET, they don't have to thaw ALL of them. So, the first group that was thawed was a group of four. But only one or two made it through the thaw process. So, they thawed a group of two and only one of those made it through. They had two embryos good to go. So, they thawed another group of four and all of them came through fine. So now we had six embryos; some had better development than others did, but they were all considered to be active.

She explained that frozen embryos don't always make it through the thaw process very well. So we were down ten frozen embryos, but had six good candidates. She recommended that we implant all six of these embryos. The odds of frozen embryos attaching were lower than fresh embryos, because of the freeze-thaw process. According to www.ivf.com, on average, 15% of fresh eight-cell embryos will implant after being transferred, but as few as 50% of embryos survive the thaw process. Ron and I were OK with the decision to implant six. All it could do was increase our chances for a successful pregnancy. And after all that time, we would be happy to welcome multiples.

After we discussed the embryos, I laid back on the table and got comfortable. Everything was very much as I expected. My doctor fussed to get the catheter around my cervix (as usual) and into the uterus. After that, the lab technicians came in with the embryos and our future children were inserted into the uterus via the catheter while being monitored by ultrasound. It sounds nice and easy, but we did have the same difficulties as the last transfer in April. My abdomen was sore, they had to push down on it to get the catheter in, and the ultrasound wand was used externally again to see where the fluid with the embryos were placed in the uterus.

But I made it through.

I had to rest on the table for about 20 minutes after the procedure, then Ron assisted me out of the room to the car. The doctor made sure to remind me to continue the progesterone oil shots every night for the next two weeks and asked me to come back for a pregnancy blood test in 14 days.

I don't think I ever laid around so much before in my life. I watched a lot of movies and slept a great deal during this time. I spent most of my time on the sofa with pillows propped up under my butt and thighs. I didn't know if this would honestly help or not, but with the laws of gravity, it made sense to me. Any extra effort that I could do to help our embryos stay in there, I was going to do.

Unfortunately, I may have received an "A" for effort, but it all proved disappointing in the end. I went in for the blood test on June 22, exactly two weeks after the FET, and the beta level was 0. I was crushed and humbled by the entire experience. And emotionally drained. Now what were we going to do? Was I destined to never bear children? I was pretty convinced that this was the case. I began to move toward just accepting that as the conclusion and moving on with our lives. Our thoughts returned to adoption again. Wondering if we could even afford to adopt now? These were the questions running through my mind. Ron and I had talked about adopting before and our hearts were open to it, but we wanted to exhaust all other measures first. We had been told that we were still good candidates for achieving a successful pregnancy, but each negative result was getting harder and harder to endure. Each treatment brought such disappointment that it left me more discouraged than when we began. If we only knew how to achieve a successful pregnancy...

Cycle # 20 – Summary

CD 1	2mg Estrace
CD 2	2mg Estrace
CD 3	2mg Estrace
CD 4	2mg Estrace
CD 5	2mg Estrace
CD 6	2mg Estrace
CD 7	2mg Estrace
CD 8	6mg Estrace
CD 9	6mg Estrace
CD 10	6mg Estrace
CD 11	2mg Estrace, 2cc Progesterone Oil
CD 12	2mg Estrace, 2cc Progesterone Oil
CD 13	2mg Estrace, 2cc Progesterone Oil
CD 14	2mg Estrace, 2cc Progesterone Oil
CD 15	2mg Estrace, 2cc Progesterone Oil, Valium, Frozen Embryo Transfer
CD 16-29	2cc Progesterone Oil

Full of Questions – Medical Leave Research

June - September 1999

It was fortunate that I had been approved for four weeks of medical leave. I needed the additional two weeks after the pregnancy results to recover emotionally before I went back to work. I needed time to be sad and grieve for my lost embryos. I prayed and prayed for the strength to see us through this difficult time. I just wanted the hurt to end, but I didn't know how to make that happen.

It was now the end of June, so I spent a lot of time outdoors in my garden. For me, gardening is very therapeutic. I am alone with the elements, and the effects of sunshine are very uplifting for me. I spent a great deal of this time in silence and taking in everything around me. Thank goodness my treatment wasn't in the dead of winter; I would have been bored and even more depressed being cooped up inside the house.

I also spent a great deal of my time off on the Internet and going to the library. I felt that it was about time that I take some direction in teaching myself more about the medical terms that I had heard during treatment. I tried to do research on anything I could find about Polycystic Ovary Syndrome. The term was used a lot when discussing my ovaries, but I didn't really have a good handle on what the syndrome was about. The library did not have anything applicable to PCOS, but there were books on many other variations of infertility. It seemed as if PCOS was so new that the only information was scattered around the Internet. I am happy to be able to say now that this was the beginning of the end for me!

While surfing the Net, I discovered a couple of websites dedicated to infertility and some dedicated to PCOS. See **Appendix D**. These sites had a great deal of information available. I was devouring all that I could. It was remarkable to read about similar circumstances. Within these websites, there were message boards allowing people to post messages and if anyone reading had an answer, they could respond. I spent a lot of time reading what people posted. As I continued to read, I discovered some new terms that I had not heard of before. For instance, IR (insulin resistance), fasting insulin blood levels, insulin-sensitizing drugs such as Metformin and Glucophage™, and discussions about specific diets. Within the www.inciid.org website, I found a bulletin board dedicated to PCOS. This was *very* nice, considering that I had not had an opportunity to draw information from others with the same diagnosis. I immediately noticed again, though, that I was a minority when it came to the symptoms that described PCOS. It has several factors to it, but on an introductory level, it is a disorder that results from abnormal levels of certain hormones. According to www.pcosupport.org the following are the symptoms to look for:

- Acanthosis Nigricans or light brown to black, rough areas of skin
- Acne
- Acrochordons or skin tags which are teardrop-shaped pieces of skin
- Amenorrhea or the absence of a menstrual cycle

- Androgenic Alopecia or male-patterned baldness
- Anovulation or the absence of ovulation
- Depression
- Hirsutism or excessive hair growth on the body
- Hyperinsulinemia or a higher than normal amount of insulin
- Infertility
- Insulin Resistance or the failure of the body to respond properly to the insulin produced by the pancreas
- Obesity or an abnormal excess of fat
- Oligomenorrhea or light and infrequent menstrual flow
- Polycystic ovaries or the presence of numerous cysts within the ovary producing a "string of pearls" like appearance on ultrasound
- Weight gain

I had polycystic ovaries, amenorrhea, anovulation, infertility and not yet diagnosed insulin resistance. The significance of these symptoms is that they can help identify the syndrome. A person with PCOS can have one or all of the symptoms that are commonly caused by hormonal irregularities of the endocrine system. The websites were particularly helpful with terminology. If I came across a new term, I could usually find it within the websites listed.

As I read through question after question, it seemed that many people were taking a fasting insulin test[18], and if it was high enough, they were taking medication that specifically targeted the breakdown of the high insulin levels. How was this related to PCOS? I kept reading.

Some women were on drugs called Metformin or Glucophage™ and, after a period of time, started to ovulate on their own again, WITHOUT the use of fertility drugs. This was interesting to me. Along with these drugs they were taking, they were learning how to eat all over again, through a low-carbohydrate, high protein diet. This type of diet was helping to keep their insulin levels down. How? I didn't know yet. They were sharing recipes, cooking tips, and talking about "SugarBusters," "The Zone," and "Dr. Atkins." I did a web search on these new terms and it pulled up www.amazon.com, which listed these as dietary books. Hmmm. What did this have to do with PCOS? I made a trip to one of our bookstores in the area that is pretty well-stocked with current publishings. There, in the diet/cookbook section, were all three of these books. Plus, I found an additional one called "Protein Power." So I read the introduction on each of them and got a general idea of the theory behind this kind of "diet" program.

Each book, in its own way, explained what the effect of foods with high doses of sugar has on our bodies. Sugar is the fuel our body needs to generate energy! When we eat foods with sugar or carbohydrates, they are broken down into glucose, which raises our blood sugar level. Insulin is then secreted from the pancreas to lower the blood sugar. Insulin acts as the mediator by lowering the

---

[18]   Fasting insulin test – A sample of blood taken in the morning after fasting since midnight the day before.

blood sugar level to within a range of 60-150 mg/dl. But, in the process, insulin promotes the storage of fat and triggers the liver to increase the production of cholesterol. Therefore, this leads to weight gain or retention and high cholesterol levels. However, when a protein-rich meal is consumed, glucogen is released from the pancreas and it promotes the mobilization of previously stored fat, therefore resulting in weight loss.

What all of this had to do with my infertility was not clear to me yet. However, I am genetically predisposed for diabetes. My maternal grandmother and my mother's sister both have diabetes.

I didn't buy any of the books because I wasn't sure that this was for me yet. But, I bought the grocery store pocket-guide to "SugarBusters," for about $5. It points out foods that are approved or not approved for this type of diet, by category. So for example, when you are shopping for fruit you can look up what is an "approved" fruit.

While doing my research, I was stacking up questions for my doctor. What was my fasting insulin ratio? Could it impact my treatment? If it was high, could I use the insulin-sensitizing drugs to lower it? Should I be on this "low-carbohydrate diet?" What did this have to do with some women getting pregnant? Why was insulin a key to their treatments? What did this have to do with PCOS?

I knew I would have to wait awhile before I could ask my questions. My doctor was having difficulty with her own pregnancy. She was in her eighth month, on bed rest, and would be on maternity leave for six weeks after the baby came. This was understandable. This meant that we needed to wait until her return to begin treatment again.

In the meantime, I went back to work and continued my online research. CD 30 approached and I had not started my period. Surprise! Surprise! I reported in with the nurses at the doctor's office and they said they would contact Dr. Gold at home to see if I could take Provera™ to induce a period. She approved the prescription and I took it for ten days. Just like clockwork, two days after I stopped Provera™ I started my period. It was August 1, 1999, a date that I will always remember as the beginning of the end.

I took it upon myself on the very same day to give the low-carb, high-protein diet a try. We weren't quite sure what kind of treatments we were going to do in the future, but it couldn't possibly hurt my chances. I didn't even know what my fasting insulin was at the time or historically.

I wasn't following the strict Dr. Atkins diet, which restricts carbohydrates completely for the first two weeks, and then introduces a strict plan of re-entering carbs gradually. I just followed a general rule of thumb that I made up. I allowed small or no portions of carbs, and larger portions of protein foods. For example, if we were having grilled steak, sweet corn on the cob, and a pasta dish, I would eat all my portion of steak, about three bites of pasta, and no corn. (What a sacrifice!) Sometimes I would make an extra dish of vegetables, such as broccoli, that were an "approved" vegetable. The hardest foods to give up, for me, were breads (rolls, breadsticks, muffins, bagels) and potatoes (mashed, baked, fried, french fries). Those were killer sacrifices for me. Otherwise, I seemed to be able to stay away from the simple sugars (sweets, candy, soda pop) very easily. It is also important to continue to eat fruit to prevent certain vitamin deficiencies, even though they contain fructose[19]. I like a wide variety of fruits, but I knew that some were off limits according to the "SugarBusters" handbook. I tried to focus on the "approved" fruits that I liked and were available to me. My favorites were those in the berry family such as raspberries, strawberries, and blueberries.

After the menu at home got a little repetitive, I went back to the bookstore. I wanted to look in the cookbook section for any "low-carb, high-protein" recipe books. Nothing (keep in mind that this was 1999, and before everyone caught on to the "Atkins" craze). Everything focused on LOW FAT. So I thought maybe a cookbook for diabetics. Nothing. I looked a little harder, and found one book called "The Low-Carb Cookbook" by Fran McCoullough. I opened to the beginning and read the Preface. She was a long-time sufferer of weight-gain even when low-fat dieting. She put together her link to insulin and carbs, changed her eating habits, and it resulted in weight loss. I looked at some of the recipes and, not only did they sound good, they looked easy to make. So I bought the book, hoping to add some variety to our low-carb cooking practices.

It seemed to me to be pretty ironic that most of my life I had been "taught" how to be a low-fat eater. The medical industry continually states that in order to stay healthy we need to watch our weight, cholesterol and blood pressure, and we can keep each of them in balance by exercising and eating a low-fat diet. "Low-fat" had just become so ingrained in my thoughts about food, it never occurred to me that I was doing my body an injustice, by *only* focusing on fat grams.

I discovered that eating a low-fat baked potato with light margarine was probably sending my glucose and insulin to astronomic levels, not to mention what my favorite breakfast meal of bagels and cream cheese was doing.

This was a pretty busy time for me: not only was I working on a new way of eating, I was also researching the option of appealing my medical insurance company for the right to cover my IVF procedure I had earlier in the year. I did most of the research for my dispute letter during my disability leave in June. The websites that I highlighted previously was where I got the idea to dispute the insurance coverage with my employer. I found some other patients online that had been willing to argue their case. Some won and some did not. Why shouldn't I try? It couldn't hurt. I felt that if I didn't try, I would never know. If I won, great! That may open the door for future infertility coverage by our employer. I wasn't recommending that our employer take on the entire financial burden of infertility treatment, but I was recommending a certain number of IVF attempts, or a "lifetime limit" in dollars. After lifetime limits had been surpassed, the benefit would expire.

I asked Dr. Gold to review the letter for her input or any comments. She said that she thought that it was very well orchestrated and wanted to know the results of the dispute. She said she had other patients that were trying to achieve similar results. My employer was privately-insured and had a process to appeal the denial

---

[19]   Fructose – a natural sugar found in fruits.

of benefits. I followed their instructions and sent my letter to the Appeals Board on September 10, 1999. I thought that I had a well-proven case for infertility patients. I could only hope that that letter was the opening to a different frame of mind for insurance companies regarding infertility treatment. I was very excited about the prospects of giving other fertility patients the ability to make the decision process easier by not concerning themselves with out-of-pocket costs. For those readers that are interested, I've included the letter in **Appendix E**. (For confidentiality purposes, the employer's name has been omitted from the text).

I returned to Dr. Gold promptly after she returned from her maternity leave. It was now early September of 1999. Our first appointment was a consultation to discuss what our next course of treatment should be, and I had a chance to ask her all of my new questions. Ron and I thought we should try another FET, since we had been fortunate to have so many embryos fertilize in April during our first IVF. We had seventeen embryos still at the lab, and the cost of another FET ($750) was minimal compared to the cost of the previous IVF ($4200). She agreed with us and we proceeded.

I started drug therapy again with estrace pills, progesterone oil, and Lupron™ injections to get my body prepared for the next transfer of embryos. However, Dr. Gold had one more new thing she wanted to add: estrogen patches. She prescribed 8 mg estrogen patches and explained when I would need to use them. I needed to start taking Lupron™ immediately, but I had to have my E2 level checked first, before we started any estrace.

After we discussed the medications, I had the opportunity to ask my questions. First and foremost, have we ever tested my fasting insulin level? She looked in my file for the bloodwork results from when I first transferred to her clinic in October of 1997, two years prior. It listed my fasting insulin ratio at 12.5 uIU/ml (international units per milliliter). She said that it was not a number that was outrageous, and that is probably why it was never focused upon. I said that everything I was reading about fasting insulin said that 3-5 uIU/ml was average or normal and anything higher was out of range. She went on to say that many of her patients that had ovaries that looked like my ovaries, had fasting insulin levels 20[20] uIU/ml and higher, and that other patients with levels near mine had successfully achieved pregnancies in the past. So I asked if it would hurt to get my fasting insulin tested again to see what it was now. I told her that I started my own version of low-carb on August 1, about six weeks prior. She responded that it couldn't hurt, and she would run a full blood screen.

I also asked, "what does Lupron™ do <u>exactly?</u>" She told me that it directly effects the pituitary gland by reducing LH levels and preventing an unwanted mid-cycle LH surge. I had read about testing the LH to FsH ratios through a blood test, to diagnose hormonal imbalances. I read that anything 3:1 or higher

---

[20]   According to <u>PCOS: The Hidden Epidemic</u>, Thatcher, Samuel S., M.D., PhD
        "There can be considerable variability between the various assays and there has
        been no central standardization. There is also considerable discrepancy about what
        constitutes abnormally high insulin".

was abnormal, and could pose a problem, so I asked why we didn't test for that. She said that it is very hard to catch the imbalance of LH to FsH in a blood test, because the LH surge has a very short life with high peaks. The FsH has a much longer life and steady. There is a low chance of catching the right moment for this particular blood test.

When I asked about the insulin-lowering drugs (Metformin/Glucophage™), she discouraged me from trying them at that point, and so did all the nurses. They said that I should find out my current insulin test results first, to see if the diet was working. They described many of the same side effects that I had read about online, mostly nausea, intestinal cramps, and severe diarrhea. I agreed that it all sounded nasty to me, but I would try it if I needed to. It couldn't be any harder than everything else that I had already been through. So we agreed to wait and see what my fasting insulin level came back at.

I had blood drawn for my E2 level after I left the doctor office. I couldn't do the fasting insulin blood test at the same time because I didn't fast beforehand. So they gave me a blood lab slip ordering the fasting insulin test for the next day. I noticed on the lab slip that she also ordered fasting glucose and TSH levels. TSH is thyroid stimulating hormone and I don't know much about it. My E2 came back at 57 and once again we were looking for that number to be under 50. I stopped in at the blood lab the next morning on my way to work. My TSH level came back at 1.09 and my Glucose was 82 mg/dL, which were within the normal ranges. It took several days to get the results of the insulin test. While we waited for the insulin test results, I stayed on the Lupron™ and was to go back for another E2 level test in one week.

Hurray! Something to cheer about. The insulin level came back at an amazing 5.3. That was much, much lower than the 12.5, but admittedly the 12.5 was from 2 years prior. My eating habits had always been consistent over the previous 2 years though, so I believe that my level prior to starting the low-carb diet on August 1 was probably quite high. So, by reaching a much lower insulin level through diet, I had no reason to use the insulin-lowering drugs. Yay!

I returned once again, one week later for my repeat E2 level blood test. It came back at 43, which was the green light to begin treatment for FET #2.

Cycle # 21 – Frozen Embryo Transfer #2

September 1999 – October 1999

I had already been on Lupron™ for 23 days and once we received the green light, I added the 2 mg estrace pill for seven days, then three 2 mg estrace pills for three days and returned to the doctor.

I went to the doctor's office for my ultrasound on September 24. She looked at the endometrial lining and measured its thickness. It was only at 7 mm; I had a little further to go. The lining is pictured in Figure D below. Because the estrace pills weren't as effective on me, Dr. Gold added estrogen patches. My new instructions were to continue the Lupron™, 6 mg of estrace pills <u>AND</u> add the estrogen patches for the next four days.

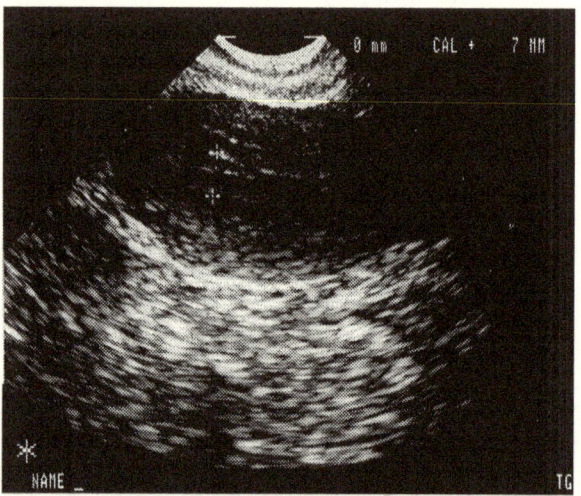

Figure D – Endometrium Lining 7 mm

The estrogen patches were in 8 mg doses. My instructions were to put one on one butt cheek and then, 12 hours later, add another one to the other butt cheek. I had to change each patch after it had been on for 24 hours.

Boy, was I on FIRE! I was unstoppable. So much estrogen, so little time! My energy and concentration levels were at an all-time high.

I went back four days later for another ultrasound, and the endometrial lining measured 13 mm. How about that? Just like magic. She also looked at my ovaries and said that they were a little enlarged, but no meaningful cysts were present. Everything looked very good. We scheduled the FET for noon two days later. We agreed to thaw the embryos until we got four NICE-looking blastocysts.

At that visit, I was given instructions to stop the Lupron™, stay on the 6 mg of estrace pills, and add a 2 cc injection of progesterone oil.

Since our FET was scheduled for 12:00 noon, I made arrangements with my friend, Denise, to drop me off on our lunch hour. I was not allowed to drive myself because I had to take a Valium one hour before the procedure. As she dropped me off, she said she'd pray for us. I told her we appreciated every bit of her prayers.

I waited until Ron arrived at the doctor's office before I went back to the procedure room. We got to watch the embryos on video again, just like the previous times, and we received photos of seven of the embryos (our very first scrapbook photos). Then our doctor reviewed the results from the lab with us. We had seventeen frozen embryos remaining when they began that morning. The lab had to thaw ALL seventeen in order to get eight that made it through the thaw. One had begun to divide already, and seven had at least one cell. They were initially frozen on day three, so they were still considered zygotes and not embryos. It is on approximately day five when they become blastocysts, and this is usually when they hatch from their wall of protein (zona pellucita) and attach themselves to the uterine lining.

Dr. Gold had a difficult time (as usual) getting the catheter around the curve in my cervix. I remember trying to imagine thoughts of Ron and me walking along a beach, holding our children's hands; splashing through the water and picking up seashells. My intent was to keep my body relaxed by focusing on these other thoughts. The more relaxed my body was, the greater the chance that the doctor could get in and out quickly. A resident doctor was assisting that day. She had to push the external ultrasound wand so hard against my pelvic area, I was sure I would develop a bruise. But it wasn't nearly as painful as it was in April when the ultrasound wand was pushed against my pelvic area which was already extremely swollen from the egg retrieval process.

Donna (my nurse) was also pushing down on my abdomen below my belly button in order to try and tilt the uterus down, so that Dr. Gold could get the catheter in. This was probably the longest it ever took to get the catheter in. It was probably about 20-25 minutes, and my doctor had to keep adjusting the speculum. After the catheter was finally in, it took virtually no time at all to insert the embryos. They finished up about 2:00 p.m. and I had to lie there for roughly two hours.

Ron came in to my room and worked on his laptop while I tried to rest and relax. I wasn't even permitted to move my legs. If I wanted to be adjusted, they came in and did it for me. At approximately 4:15 p.m., I got up from the table and got dressed. We stepped out into the hall and paid the $750 for the cost of the FET. Everyone wished us well, and I said that I'd see them in two weeks for the pregnancy test. I was told to continue taking the 6 mg of estrace pills, the 2 cc injection of progesterone oil, and one prenatal vitamin each day for the next two weeks.

Ron and I had scheduled a vacation to New York City and a Connecticut bed and breakfast prior to knowing about the dates of the FET treatment. The timing worked out perfectly, and we spent the next week relaxing on our trip. Unfortunately, the only drawback for Ron was that I was not allowed to drive. So I got to admire all the beautiful fall scenery in Connecticut and New York while Ron drove. It was a very relaxing trip. We were able to reconnect with each other again, without the distraction of work or our home life. We passed the driving time by picking out baby names that we liked. We had chosen 3 possible girl names and 2 boy names by the end of our trip. Since we had previously scheduled a week off of work on vacation, I didn't file for a medical leave for this treatment cycle.

I had about five more days to wait until "the blood test," and I couldn't wait any longer. I went ahead and calculated the approximate due date for this baby. On or around June 23, 2000 is what I came up with. Uh-oh, now I had created an emotional connection to this pregnancy. I did it again! Even after all that I've learned, I keep setting myself up.

It was about two days before the test and I felt as if my breasts were more tender than usual. But because I had been deceived before, I was always so skeptical to interpret how I was feeling. I didn't want to let that happen again. Maybe these were just signs of my oncoming menstrual cycle?

On Friday, October 15, I had my blood drawn at 8:30 a.m. and then went on to work. Even the ladies in the blood lab knew me by then and why I was there, especially Rose. I always ended up at her station. She always wished me good luck and hoped I wouldn't have to come back, because that, of course, meant that I would be pregnant!

When I arrived at work that day, I had to focus my attention on an enormous project that I had been working on for months. We were in the middle of launching a major debt issuance program. We had been working intensely on this project for the previous two months, and the timing was unbelievable. On one hand, I was satisfied professionally because I thoroughly enjoyed what I had learned and what we had accomplished, but at the same time personally, I was just a wreck. I had been entrenched in treatment for so long during the last three years, I was drained both emotionally and physically.

Cycle # 21 – Summary

CD 1	2mg Estrace, Lupron™
CD 2	2mg Estrace, Lupron™
CD 3	2mg Estrace, Lupron™
CD 4	2mg Estrace, Lupron™
CD 5	2mg Estrace, Lupron™
CD 6	2mg Estrace, Lupron™
CD 7	2mg Estrace,Lupron™
CD 8	6mg Estrace, Lupron™
CD 9	6mg Estrace Lupron™
CD 10	6mg Estrace Lupron™, ultrasound
CD 11	6mg Estrace, Lupron™ Estrogen patches
CD 12	6mg Estrace, Lupron™ Estrogen patches
CD 13	6mg Estrace, Lupron™ Estrogen patches
CD 14	6mg Estrace, Lupron™ Estrogen patches, ultrasound
CD 25	Frozen Embryo Transfer
CD 17-33	6 mg Estrace, 2cc Progesterone Oil, 1 pre-natal vitamin

What now?

When I didn't hear from the doctor by 11:30 a.m., I called them. Sandy picked up the phone. After I told her who it was, she said, "I'm so sorry, Amy. It was negative. Dr. Gold was disappointed too."

After you hear those words, it is hard to speak. I just focused on trying not to burst out crying so that I could finish the phone conversation.

Sandy said, "I know that you are heartbroken."

I guess that is one way of putting it. I was so very sad. Again. When will it ever end?

I asked Sandy to ask if Dr. Gold would call me later at home when she had a moment. I needed to talk in depth about our prognosis.

I beeped Ron, who was unreachable by phone because he was on a job site. I waited for his return call. When I picked up the phone, he said, "What's up, hon?"

"It was negative..."

"Oh no. Are you okay?"

"I'll be alright..." My voice fading off.

"Why don't you go home and get some rest. I'll come right home after I'm done out here."

"I was thinking about doing that anyway. Dr. Gold is going to call me at home later on. I want to be there to receive her call. I'll see you at home tonight. Love you."

"Love you too."

I left work that day at 12:30 p.m. and cried all the way home. Once I got home, I cried myself to sleep. I was pretty convinced that it was all over for us. We had no options left to achieve a pregnancy, and I was at the end of my emotional rope. If IVF and FET wouldn't work, what else was there? I tried so hard to keep myself together; I didn't want to spiral down into a depressive, altered state of being, but I was so sad... I think I tried to convince myself that I could accept defeat and get past this, but it is so hard.

At this point, you may wonder why having a baby was just so important to me. After enduring this emotional and physical battleground, why did I feel the need to persist on? I am not really sure. As I look back, I try to pinpoint what drove my desire to want to become a parent. Was it the social influence to have children, the responsibility felt to contribute to our society, or an intimate expression of love shared between two people – the greatest gift of establishing a family.

I think it was a mixture of many of these. First, I think most of us grow up assuming that we (women) can have children, not *will* have children, but at least *can* have children. Sort of a birthright. Having children is not something that I thought about continuously growing up nor did it shape my future and direction in life. I was not one to say, "I want to grow up to be a mom and raise 5 kids." It was secondary to finding my way through relationships, education and career.

Although I did always envision my life in the nucleus family, having two parents and, at some point, kids.

Once we settled into our life together, it seemed the next logical step. Was it the next logical step because that is what society or everyone else does? Or was it another goal on a list that Type A's have? Or would it be proof of the most intimate level of sharing that a relationship could achieve, two people creating a third. According to Expecting Miracles, by Dr. Christo Zouves, "it is the nature of living things to reproduce."

As I matured and evolved into a woman with goals and direction, I naturally reached the next level. The next level for us was to have a child together, create a family, experience the responsibility of raising a new human being. The love and relationship that I shared with my husband was such a part of my being, that I wanted to experience parenthood with him. The honor of "training" a human being to become a functioning participant in society, is in fact one of our greatest gifts to our society. And of course, without children, there is no future.

I know that at one point I told my friend Denise that I must be at fault for obsessing about this dream. She said that it was perfectly normal to dream about becoming a mother and having a family, I shouldn't feel bad about it. Most people don't have to work this hard to become parents. The disadvantage to my Type A personality is that no matter how hard I worked and no matter what I did, I could not do this alone. I was dependent on the help of others to achieve a pregnancy.

Dr. Gold's phone call that afternoon woke me up. I had prepared a couple of questions prior to her call that I wanted to go over with her. She was very supportive and considerate. Her tone was very calming and patient. I didn't know if any other patients asked as many questions as I always did, but she never seemed to mind. I wanted to be as proactive as I could in my treatment.

My first question was "am I medically capable of carrying a child through a pregnancy?" She said, "Yes!" There was nothing that she had seen thus far that would lead her to believe otherwise. Next I asked, "Did the one-cell embryos that were transplanted even have a chance?" She confessed that she thought that just the one embryo that had started to divide had a really good chance. And she commented that all my previous embryos were produced with eggs from when I had a much higher insulin level earlier in the year. There were studies being done that addressed egg quality and uterine lining quality under high insulin levels. Hmmm. Could that have played a major role in all of our frozen embryos? They may not have ever had a chance. Embryo quality is the leading factor in my losing the cycle when I took too much Profasi™ and had OHSS.

She asked if I knew if my mother had taken a medication called DES to prevent a miscarriage when she was pregnant with me. I wasn't sure, but I told her I was 99% certain that she had not. When I asked why, she said that the long-term effects of that drug on the baby girls that were born are related to some infertility cases. But I didn't fit that profile.

I asked if we should go through another IVF process, but transplant the embryos at day five instead of day three. This would allow us to choose the strongest embryos for successful implantation. I can't remember the reason Dr. Gold gave me, but I know she discouraged the five-day embryo transplant.

We went on to have a very good, thorough conversation about my history and prognosis. We talked a lot about the effects of insulin and most of the other findings that we had learned up to that point about my body. One good point about the IVF procedure was that it proved that my eggs and Ron's sperm **were** compatible together. They did fertilize well, *and* at a high percentage rate. This was something that we did not know prior to the IVF, because we had always performed IUI's.

All I had left was one final question. What would she do, if she were me? During our conversation, I had made a suggestion that maybe we should try a couple more ovulation induction cycles with an IUI, now that my insulin level was much lower. Maybe this would improve the condition of the eggs and possible embryos in addition to improving the quality of the uterine lining. This was also the less expensive option, as compared to the IVF procedure. Dr. Gold said that she would probably make the same decision that I had suggested. And she said that my lower insulin level, would probably improve the effectiveness of the Fertinex™ (FsH) injections.

So that is what we decided to do. At the end of our conversation, she asked if I had ever had an HSG (hysterosalpinogram) performed. I told her I didn't think so, because I had never even heard of it before. She said that I would remember if I did. She explained that it is a method to check to see if the fallopian tubes are open. Any blockages would indicate that an egg could not reach the uterus. She wanted me to schedule an HSG test at the hospital, ten days after the onset of my period from this cycle. This would allow her to verify that the fallopian tubes were in fact open and that an egg could reach the uterus with no difficulty.

Now, I was a bit surprised that this had not been brought up before. What if they had been blocked for years? Then all those prior ovulation induction cycles and IUI's never would have even had a chance? Maybe the sperm and egg never even met in the fallopian tubes?

She also started me on Lupron™ again right away. I was to call the office as soon as my period started in order to schedule the HSG and an E2 blood test. When her office called in the prescription for Lupron™, they also called in Diazipan (Valium), Ibuprofen, and Vicadin (similar to Percocet) for the day of the HSG procedure.

Ron and I also decided at that time, that if I wasn't pregnant by the end of the year (it was then October), we'd move on to the possibility of adopting a child. In my spare time I researched international adoptions on the Internet.

I received my response that month from my employer's Heath Insurance Appeals Board. The letter outlined why my infertility treatment was denied by quoting from the "Uncovered Benefits" section out of the Benefits Manual. I was going to need to re-submit my letter and arguments again if I wanted to challenge this level of coverage by trying to change the policy. Therefore, I re-submitted my original letter and supporting documentation again for another round of waiting.

Cycle 22 – Success at Last

October 1999 – November 1999

I had a "Big Time" period start just five days after the negative pregnancy results. I would imagine that my uterine lining was pretty thick preparing for the FET. I called the doctor's office to report the onset of menses and scheduled the HSG and E2 blood test for one week later.

The Hysterosalpinogram

On the day of my HSG, I remember what an incredibly beautiful October day it was. The air was crisp and smelled of fall, the sun was bright, and the trees were dressed in their fall colors. Ron dropped me off at work in the morning this time so that my vehicle stayed home. I had already made arrangements with my friend, Rose, to drop me off at the hospital on our lunch hour. I scheduled that afternoon off as vacation time, and Ron would pick me up at the hospital when the procedure was completed.

By this time in my treatment history, I was keeping track of all my visits, blood tests, prescriptions, and results. But during the previous month, I had started keeping a journal of my feelings, emotions, and frustrations. In this journal, I had been working on a poem that expressed what I thought it would feel like, to be a parent. Just before I went to the hospital for the HSG, I finished it.

The Gift of Life

The day has finally arrived
That you come home to me,
So small, fragile and beautiful
A small miracle to see.

A little one so innocent
So peaceful and so dear,
We are parent and child forever now
So blessed that you are here.

Tiny fingers, feet and toes
A personality that is your own,
The newest gift from heaven
And we get to take you home.

As I talk to you today
My expressions make you smile,
Eyes wide with wonder
Let's hold this moment for a while.

And when I look down at you
Curled up in my arm,
I promise to teach and guide you
And protect you from harm.

Your room smells of baby powder
And the lullabies are playing,
We thought this day would never come
I am sure the angels are saying...

"You see, miracles can happen
When there is hope and you believe,
That His love will be the strength to guide you
We are not alone, He doesn't leave."

We know our time is limited
For you will grow and need to explore,
The world and all its mysteries
We couldn't offer you more.

Now my mind shifts back to the present
And I realize that I've done it again,
You see, we live each day with Infertility
And I pray, "God give me the strength to get through this. Amen!"

So some day we will meet you,
We'll hold you, and hug you,
We'll tuck you in warmly
And of course we will Love You!

For there is no greater gift
For a man and wife,
Than the birth of their child
The gift of life.

I read this poem to Rose while driving to the hospital, and we were sobbing by the time I finished reading it. When we pulled up to the entrance doors, she wished me all God's blessings and she said, "Good things happen to good people." I told her that I'd call her later and let her know how I was doing.

When I arrived at the hospital, I checked in at the desk in the X-ray area for the HSG, then I went to the lab to get my blood work drawn for my E2 level. The blood test was fast and easy, nothing out of the ordinary. Then I proceeded back to the X-ray waiting room.

Once again, I had to take a Diazipan (Valium generic) one hour before the surgery time. This pill was supposed to take a little bit of the edge off and make me relax. I took it just before we left work on our way to the hospital.

When they called me back and took me to my room, they instructed me to take all my clothes and jewelry off in the little bathroom and put on the hospital gown. I then needed to come out and sit on the table and wait for my doctor and the nurses. The medication worked pretty well for me. I almost fell asleep lying on the table waiting for them to come in. It was very quiet...

Then everyone came through the doors together. In walked Dr. Gold, an X-ray technician, and a nurse. My doctor started the procedure by inserting the speculum to open my vagina. She then inserted a needle with some medication that she said would numb the muscles attached to the uterus and cervix. It stung, but it wasn't so bad. It felt a little like when they do an IUI, a bit of pressure, then an uncomfortable poke. Then it came time for the dye (but it is a clear liquid). Dr. Gold drew it out of a bottle with a huge syringe. While she prepared this, the X-ray technician was getting the huge machine ready. I was on what seemed like a gigantic table, and the X-ray machine arm was hanging down from the ceiling. He adjusted it so they could see my ovaries and fallopian tubes on the screen. They would need to watch the screen while the dye was being released. Once the X-ray machine was in the right position, Dr. Gold inserted the syringe and injected some of the dye on the left side, then the right side. It immediately brought tears to my eyes, because it stung. That part went pretty fast though. As the fluid filled my uterus and tubes, I felt some abdominal pressure. We all watched the screen as the fluid went all the way through the tubes. That's when they quickly took three pictures, one of the left side, one of the right side, then one full frontal that showed both tubes and ovaries on the same screen. After the X-rays were taken, Dr. Gold quickly pulled everything back out of me. Ahh... Pressure relieved.

With all the emotion attached to this test and the overall discomfort, I burst out crying. Tears were still trickling when Dr. Gold came to my side and explained that everything looked great. She described what was on the X-ray screen; the big blob was the uterus of course, and the thin fallopian tubes were visible, one on each side of the uterus. She pointed at the large area at the end of each of the fallopian tube near each ovary and she explained that this is where fertilization usually happens, before the trip down the fallopian tube.

She announced that I was all set to do another ovulation induction cycle. However, this time she wanted to try a new FsH drug called Follistim™ instead of Fertinex™ because Fertinex™ had not worked up to this point. She said that she typically prescribed Fertinex™, because it is a little bit less expensive. But she wanted to wait until she received my E2 results this afternoon before going ahead. She said she would give me a call when they came in.

I proceeded to put myself back together and got dressed. I asked the nurse if I was also allowed to get a copy of one of the X-rays. I thought it was pretty cool to see the internal view of my uterus and tubes, plus Ron had not been there to see everything. She said I'd have to pay for it, but it was only like $8. So I have my very own "picture" of my uterus and fallopian tubes. How cool!

I returned to the waiting room and hadn't been there long when Ron arrived. He picked up all my stuff for me, and we proceeded to the car.

He looked at me and asked how it went. And I quickly said, "Before or after I cried?"

He said, "It went that well, huh?" with a great deal of concern on his face.

"I suppose it wasn't that bad looking back, but it did hurt. Good thing is that everything is clear. We are good to go," I responded.

"Well, good! Let's get you home."

"Would you like to see a picture of my insides?"

"You have pictures?"

"Sure, I requested a copy of the X-ray for us. I thought it was pretty cool," I said as he rolled his eyes.

Ovulation Induction

Sandy called me later that afternoon and said that my E2 was at 10 and that I was good to start my meds. She confirmed that I was still taking my Lupron™. She said that they were going to call in 30 amps of Follistim™ and one 10 k unit of Profasi™ for me. She instructed me to take 3 Follistim™ amps for 5 days, then 2½ amps for 3 days, and return for an ultrasound and E2 blood test. That would be on November 6, 1999. I told her that we'd pick the medications up in the morning and start the taking them that evening.

I had been maintaining my low-carb diet since August 1. On November 6, the ultrasound showed many follicles on both ovaries at 14-16 mm and my E2 was 1166, perfect. "Come back in two days," they said.

I went back in on Monday, and I was a little bit more swollen on my left side than on my right. The ultrasound showed I had many follicles on both ovaries of 12-18 mm. The ultrasound is shown below as **Figure E**. My E2 was 2863. I left with instructions to take 3 amps that night and 2 amps on Tuesday night and come back in on Wednesday.

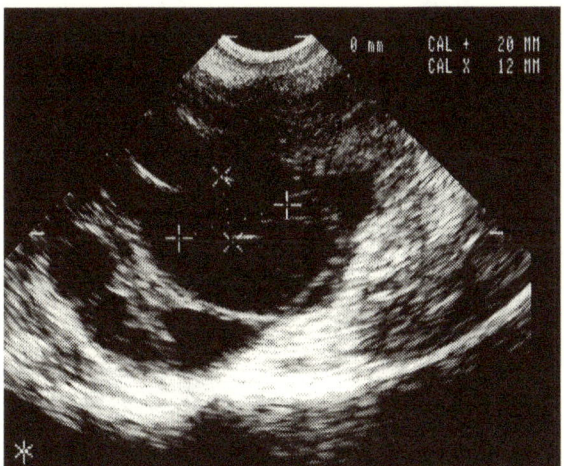

Figure E – Follicles, Cycle 22, Day 20

On Wednesday, I felt extremely full and my breasts were <u>very</u> sensitive. I went to the lab for my blood draw before work. The doctor's office called me in the afternoon and my E2 was 5236. I was told to coast that day and come back for another E2 test in the morning. Once again, just like most of the times before this, I was juggling all of these treatments before work or at lunch, trying to make sure that my time was made up at work. We were still working crazy hours putting together the offering memorandum for our debt issuance program.

I had my blood drawn on Thursday morning, and Dr. Gold called me at work that afternoon. My E2 level was 9240, it went up even without taking any meds last night, but she had told me in the past that the life of the FsH is approximately 2 days. So the FsH I took 2 days ago was still developing the follicles in the ovaries. This E2 level was way too high. She told me to coast again today and come back in the morning for another blood test.

On Friday, November 12, I had seen the doctor every day that week except for Tuesday. I went in at 7:40 a.m. for my blood draw and an ultrasound. The pictures are below in **Figure F**. Just look at all the follicles! The dark black circles are the follicles filled with fluid. Each follicle has a potential egg developing inside. Sandy called me in the afternoon with my E2 level, it was now at 11429. Once again, that was just too high.

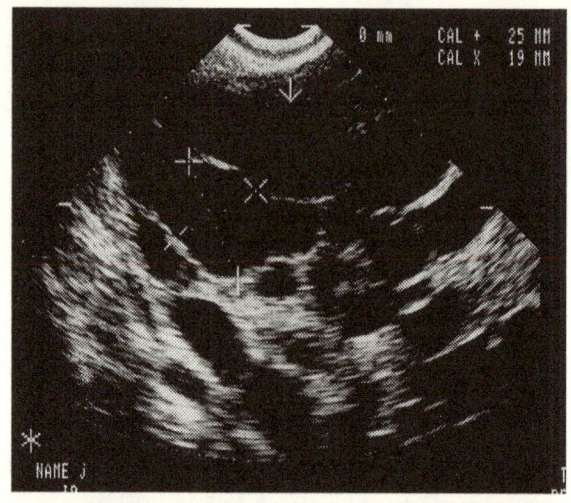

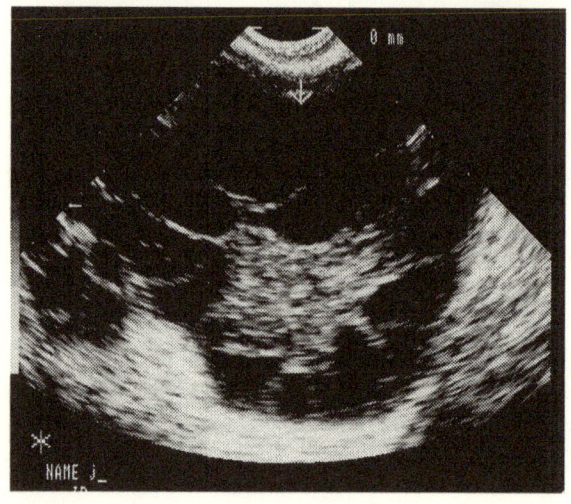

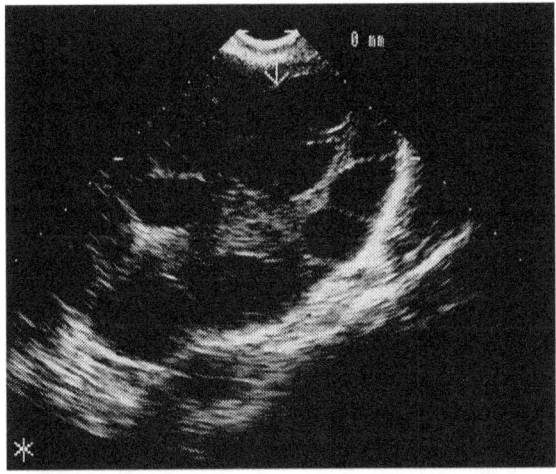

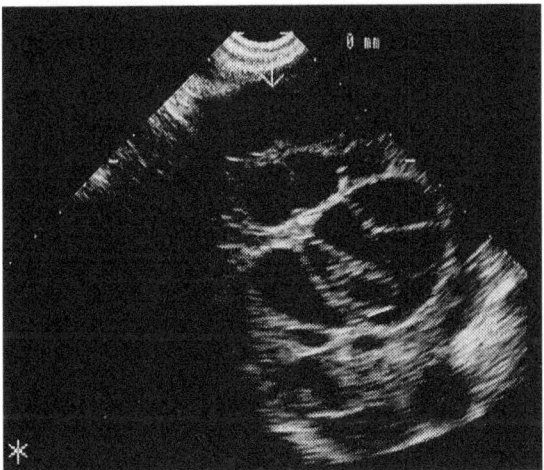

Figure F – Follicles, Cycle 22 Day 24

But then I got another call around 4:15 p.m. that day. It was Sandy again. She said that the lab called to fess up on an error that they had made. They processed the test with the wrong dilution, which gave a bad reading on the results. The new E2 level for that day was only 6252. They were not sure if yesterday's test was done correctly either. Thank goodness the lab didn't wait any longer to call, because we would have lost the cycle. Dr. Gold instructed me to take the Profasi™ shot that night at 10:00 p.m., and the IUI would be scheduled for 8:00 a.m. on Sunday morning. A sperm sample also had to be at the lab on Sunday morning by 7:00 a.m. for their shower and shave.

I was still feeling full and swollen in the abdomen area, and I was also extremely tired; just dragging and dragging. In the midst of all of this, I received the final response to my denial of benefits claim. They ultimately determined that

81

I had "exhausted my legal rights" to argue that infertility was a disease under the ADA and that they had no further responsibility to grant my request to change the coverage parameters under their plan. I have included a copy of this response letter under **Appendix F.** I was disappointed and dropped the case. I should have persisted and continued on, but the next step would have required that we hire an attorney. Although I truly believe that I had a remarkably valid claim under the ADA, at the time I was so worn down from my treatment schedule and working so many hours that I did not have the strength or the savings to continue.

IntraUterine Insemination

We got up pretty early that Sunday morning. It takes about 30 minutes to get to the doctor's office, and we had to get our showers, AND we had to have time to collect the sample. We met the lab technician at 7:00 a.m. and she whisked away Ron's sperm sample. We told her that we were going for breakfast, and we'd be back by 8:00 a.m. She said that she may be gone by then, but the doctor would be there. In one small twist in all of this, Dr. Gold was going to be in Washington D.C. that week, and could not perform our IUI, therefore, her partner Dr. Waters would be performing this one.

When we returned from breakfast, Sandy met us in the waiting room and told us to come on back. Everything was ready. Dr. Waters came in and explained what he'd be doing. But we already knew. We had survived other attempts.

Everything started out very much the same. He inserted the speculum and tried to guide the catheter up around my cervix into the uterus. He attempted many times, but it just wouldn't go in. We had warned him how difficult it had been in the past to do this. Then the next thing I know, I felt an incredibly painful, pinching feeling deep inside. It instantly brought tears to my eyes and my fists clenched. I looked at Ron and winced. Sandy was standing on the opposite side of me that Ron was on, and she kept asking me if I was okay. I kept nodding "yes," but it hurt so much! It seemed like forever after that, but the next attempt to guide the catheter through was successful.

Once the catheter was in, the sperm sample was drawn up in the syringe and inserted into my uterus through the catheter. That was it. He then took out the catheter and the speculum. They lifted my legs onto the table and told me to relax for about 20 minutes.

After Dr. Waters left the room, I asked Sandy, "What the hell hurt so much?"

She said that he used an instrument that helped straighten out the cervix. It was called a tenaculum[21]. She described it as looking somewhat like a clamp on a long handle, but the clamp has teeth on it. My eyes must have gotten really big because she said, "I know how much it hurts. I've had one used on me before. Supposedly they say that there are no nerve endings on the cervix, but I don't

---

[21] Tenaculum – a hooked surgical instrument for grasping and holding parts during an operation. <u>Melloni's Illustrated Medical Dictionary, Fourth Ed</u>. p. 639.

believe that." I just kept saying that nothing has EVER hurt like that pinching feeling did. Ron even said that when he watched the doctor do the procedure, he thought that the tool looked like a pretty nasty instrument.

Now that that was all done, I was to rest at home and begin taking the 2 cc of progesterone oil injections. Two weeks was the timeframe to wait once again. I told Sandy I'd see her in two weeks for the pregnancy test.

Ovarian HyperStimulation Again

The IUI was on Sunday, and I only made it to Tuesday. Since I had experienced Ovarian HyperStimulation Syndrome the previous year, I knew the signs and symptoms: I began to feel nauseous by Sunday evening; I had an overwhelming feeling of pressure on my internal organs; it hurt to touch my belly area; getting up off of the couch was excruciating; I could feel my organs shift when I stood up; I felt short of breath and clammy – the abdominal swelling was putting pressure on my diaphragm resulting in my shortness of breath.

I didn't go to work until Monday afternoon, and the only reason I did go in was because I had my performance appraisal. By Monday evening, I couldn't eat, but I could still drink fluids. On Tuesday morning I decided to stay at home. But by 9:30 a.m., I paged Ron. He was at a job site that day, and I wanted to tell him that I couldn't stand the pain any more, I was going to call the doctor's office. By then, I could not keep any fluids down. I kept dry-heaving, even when I sucked on ice cubes. I generally have a high tolerance to pain. Because of my OHSS experience the year prior, I knew when I'd reached my threshold. When I couldn't keep liquids down any longer and stopped urinating, that's when I needed to be treated.

I called the doctor and talked to Sandy. She said to come in right away. She said that I would probably be admitted for OHSS.

When I called Ron back, I told him that I was going to call my mom at work to see if she could take me to the doctor and, if she wasn't available, then I would call him again. When I called my mom, she was in a meeting. I had the receptionist go ahead and interrupt her and get her on the phone. When I told her what was happening, she said that she was on her way, and it would take her about 45 minutes to get to my house. My sister-in-law came over to sit with me until my mom arrived.

I was a mess. I was crying because it hurt so much. And because I got such good response from this cycle, I didn't want to lose it and have to start all over. I just cried and cried, which made my abdomen hurt even more.

I was ready to go when my mom arrived. I grabbed my purse, tissues, and a cup to throw up in for the car ride. When we got to the doctor's office, I was taken back to a room and laid down right away. Sandy said that Dr. Waters was in surgery and Dr. Gold would be in Washington, DC until the next day. We just had to wait until Dr. Waters got back from surgery.

It didn't seem like we waited very long. He came in and quickly checked my ovaries and follicles. The ultrasound showed that the ovaries were huge; they were very swollen. He said that I would be admitted to the hospital to monitor my kidneys and control the nausea. Sandy said that they would page Dr. Gold and let her know what was happening to me. They expected her to return on Wednesday evening.

This was pretty much what I expected. Not the OHSS, but the treatment of it. This time around I wasn't as caught off guard as I was the previous year. The only difference from the first OHSS and this one, was the timing. Last time, I was inseminated on a Monday, got sick on Friday, and went to the hospital on Saturday (5 days). This time, I was inseminated on Sunday, and the swelling started immediately on Sunday night, sick on Monday, and in the hospital by Tuesday (2 days).

Mom drove me to the hospital and we proceeded to Admitting. I had requested a private room this time, because it was hard to rest last year with my roommate's activities. I was wheeled to a room and had an IV with medication administered rather quickly - the same as last time, anti-nausea and morphine for pain. Ahh, it was heaven. I was finally able to stop throwing up and get some rest. My mom stayed with me until Ron got there after work. And I as far as I remembered, I slept that entire afternoon.

I called my office on Wednesday to let everyone know what happened to me. I spoke to my brand new boss of two weeks and explained my condition. I was having a hard time speaking at length because of the abdominal pressure, so I was very brief. He said that he could tell that my breathing and speech were strained. I told him that I'd call with an update on my prognosis when I knew what was going on. He told me to concentrate on my health, and they would take care of everything at the office.

After I hung up with him, I called my voice mail to change my message. I believe that I said something like, "This is Amy Hansen and I have become extremely ill and do not have a return date. If your call needs immediate attention, please call *** at ***. I will return all other calls when I return. Thank you." I am sure this message was a bit alarming to the business associates who may have called over the next few weeks. I was hardly ever out of the office ill.

On Wednesday evening, Dr. Gold came up to the hospital to see me about 7:30 p.m. It was hard to wait all day for her to get there. I knew that she would "drain" my belly for me and relieve some of the pressure.

She hugged me as soon as she came in my room. "Are you ready for a tap?" she asked.

"I sure am," I said.

She and the nurse, Jennifer, set up to drain the peritoneal cavity, or belly area. They gathered the same supplies as before: a syringe with a numbing agent, a large needle with a catheter tube attached, iodine swabs, cotton balls, and a bucket to catch the fluid. She poked around my belly, found a good spot, numbed the area with the shot, waited a bit, then stuck the needle with the syringe into my abdomen, and started to suck on the other end like a siphon. There it goes! She pointed the catheter over the bedside, into the bucket on the floor, and we just sat and talked. As the fluid came out, I noticed that it looked to me like the color of tea. We were betting how much fluid we thought would come out, one liter, two liters?

It ended up to be 2100 cc which is about 2.3 liters. All that was just sitting in my peritoneal cavity. When she was done, I felt so much better. I could breath deeper. It's a little scary when you can only take shallow breaths. It feels as if you are suffocating. After all my research in the prior months and my experience with OHSS the previous year, I had a much better understanding of where this fluid came from[22]. It was classic OHSS.

I still had not eaten anything solid since being admitted, but I had stopped vomiting. I also had not urinated in what seemed like a very long time, 1½ days ago. On Thursday night, Dr. Gold came in around 6:45 p.m. and did another drain. This time only 1100 cc was drained, or approximately 1 liter.

By Friday, I weighed 152½, which was only 5 pounds higher than when I was at the doctor's office on Tuesday. It was a long day while I waited for Dr. Gold to get there. I felt pretty good up until about 2:00 p.m., then my belly area began to feel overwhelmingly large and very tender. When Dr. Gold arrived about 8:45 p.m., she immediately did another tap and hardly anything came out, maybe 100 cc. So they wheeled in the ultrasound unit and looked for any pockets of fluid. She couldn't find any, but she said each of my ovaries were about the size of a grapefruit. I told her that I was so uncomfortable, I would never get any sleep. She said that she could prescribe a sleeping pill for me that night and that should help me get some needed rest. It worked beautifully. I slept well until the phlebotomist came in at 6:30 a.m. to draw my blood.

On Saturday, my intake and output started to finally shift in the other direction. I think I was out of bed to urinate every two hours. This is a good indication of the beginning of the end of OHSS. I was even able to eat real food and keep it down. I had started to feel more like my normal state of being.

The blood tests on Sunday morning came back looking good, and Dr. Gold asked me how I felt. I said that I was stir crazy in the hospital after six days and was definitely ready to go home. But I knew that I was still swollen and sore. She said that pain management was really all they could do now, so she prescribed me all sorts of things to help. I had Percocet for pain, Nembutal Sodium to sleep, Promethazine for nausea and stool softeners[23]. Whoopee!

She recommended that I stay home from work that week and let my ovaries rest; they were still very much enlarged. She said that I could also be pregnant, and I may start to feel symptoms from that. I had heard that before, so I was like, "Yah, right."

That Thursday was Thanksgiving, and I took it very easy; not a lot of holiday activity for me that week, just a lot of eating and sleeping.

---

[22] PCOS: The Hidden Epidemic "OHSS – process associated with altered permeability and leakage of protein-rich fluid from the small vessels of the ovary into the pelvic, abdominal and possibly pleural (lung) cavities" pg. 382

[23] Each of these medications are safe for the embryo/fetus if pregnancy is achieved.

After the long holiday weekend, I geared myself back up for going back to work. I had been off almost two complete weeks now. Never before had I been gone that long unexpectedly.

Cycle # 22 – Summary	
CD 1-10	Lupron™ only, HsG and bloodwork
CD 11	Lupron™, 3 amps Follistim™
CD 12	Lupron™, 3 amps Follistim™
CD 13	Lupron™, 3 amps Follistim™
CD 14	Lupron™, 3 amps Follistim™
CD 15	Lupron™, 3 amps Follistim™
CD 16	Lupron™, 2½ amps Follistim™
CD 17	Lupron™, 2½ amps Follistim™
CD 18	Lupron™, 2½ amps Follistim™, ultrasound
CD 19	Lupron™, 2½ amps Follistim™
CD 20	Lupron™, 3 amps Follistim™
CD 21	Lupron™, 2 amps Follistim™
CD 22-25	Lupron™, coast
CD 26	IUI
CD 28-33	OHSS, hospital stay, progesterone oil

The Final Results

On Monday morning, I went to the blood lab around 7:30 a.m. then proceeded to work. I spent most of my morning going through e-mail, voice mail, and paper mail from my two-week absence. I knew word would get out that I was back, and the calls started coming in. It was approximately 11:00 a.m. when my phone rang.

I picked up the receiver and said, "This is Amy Hansen speaking." This was my standard answering phrase.

The female voice at the other end said, "Is this the pregnant Amy Hansen speaking?"

I don't know what was going through my foggy head at that time, but for some reason I immediately thought that this was some kind of a prank call. I couldn't believe someone would pull such a horrible stunt on me. I replied sarcastically, "Excuuuuse me?"

Then there was some shuffling commotion at the other end of the line. The person picked up the receiver and a female voice said, "Amy, this is Dr. Gold, you are pregnant!"

That's when it all clicked, and I just burst out crying. She said, "You did it, it is so your turn, you and Ron will make wonderful parents! Congratulations!"

All I could muster out between tears was "Thank you so much." Over and over again, that's all I said.

All of the other women from her office were on the speakerphone with her when she called. There was so much cheering and clapping in the background. Everyone was so excited and glad that it was finally our turn for good news.

Dr. Gold told me that the beta level was 84. That was definitely positive, but it wasn't a super high number. So she asked if I'd like to get another beta level test in two days. I said "sure, that would be no problem." Typically, the beta number will approximately double every 48 hours. Therefore, my beta level should be around 160 on Wednesday.

I sat dumbfounded for a moment after the best phone call of my life. I don't know why it didn't occur to me that the call could have been Dr. Gold. I wasn't sitting by the phone waiting for the results because I guess I just got used to getting each call after lunch, and I had learned not to anticipate and wait because it was always just a huge letdown.

So this is what it feels like. I am pregnant! I'm finally going to be a mom.

I got up and shut my office door and immediately paged Ron. He returned my call shortly thereafter. When he said, "What's up, dear?" I replied "Dr. Gold says that you're gonna be a daddy!"

"Really?" he exclaimed.

"Yes, really," I said.

"That is such great news. I can't believe it. That is great. While I was on my way to calling you back, I was trying to think of something different to say that you haven't already heard, in order to cheer you up. I figured it would have been negative."

I went on to tell him all about the conversation with Dr. Gold. We decided to send the doctor's office a dozen roses to express our thankfulness and gratitude. We just couldn't wait to see each other at home that evening.

During our phone conversation, Dr. Gold had also said that I would need to continue taking the supplemental progesterone through the first 12 weeks of the pregnancy and begin taking prenatal vitamins. I was still taking the progesterone, so we just had to pick up the vitamins.

I finally pulled myself together and walked out of my office and into Denise's office next door. I stood there for just a moment until she looked up at me, then I said in a quiet whisper so that everyone around could not hear, "The test came back positive. The doctor said that I'm pregnant."

She came around her desk, shut her door, and we hugged and cried. She had been such a pillar of strength during some of my darkest, saddest moments. She was usually the first, besides Ron, to know when I got the many other disappointing phone calls because she sat next to me. She and I sat and talked about my conversation with Dr. Gold. Then she called another friend of ours, Rose, and asked her to come by her office.

When she opened the door and walked in, she saw me sitting there. All I could do was nod my head and smile. Her eyes got really big, and she shut the door behind her. I was so choked up, I couldn't even talk. I stood up and we hugged and hugged. Luckily, we went unnoticed. I didn't want to make a scene, because I didn't want everyone else to know about this until we were past the first trimester. We had come so far, but we had so far to go yet. I didn't want to do anything that would risk the pregnancy.

I was back at the doctor office two days later for another blood test. Donna told me that she was the one that took the call from the blood lab on that Monday morning, and when the results were read she asked for them to please repeat the patient name and the beta level again. She apparently screamed down the hall to Dr. Gold, and the lab techs, Taylor and Tracy, came to see what was going on, they said "it must be Amy Hansen's results." And results it was. She said everyone was ecstatic. And that's when they all gathered to make the phone call to me.

Even the technicians in the blood lab congratulated me, especially Rose. She and I had gotten to know each other from my many trips to her station. She said that I reminded her of her daughter.

The beta level result on Wednesday did not quite double. This time it was 143, which was definitely higher than Monday's level. But Dr. Gold suggested that I come back again on Friday just to make sure. Ron and I decided that we would wait to tell our families until the blood tests were over. We really wanted to make sure that we were in the positive range before we got everyone's hopes up. Most of our family members knew that we should be getting the results soon because the insemination and OHSS was over two weeks before.

I went once again on Friday morning and it was 269. It still did not double, _but_ it was definitely higher than Wednesday's. The doctor asked if we wanted to check it again on Monday. Ron and I agreed that we were elated with the number that came back. I had never had a reading above 9 before and 269 definitely indicated that I was pregnant; that was good enough for us. So we left it at that and hoped and prayed everything would go well for this baby. Before we left the doctor's office, we scheduled a six-week ultrasound with Dr. Gold to look for the gestational sac and a heartbeat. According to the gestational calendar, I was already considered over four weeks pregnant on that Friday. In two more weeks, we would be able to see the baby's heartbeat. Dr. Gold also said that this would be when we would be able to tell how many eggs fertilized.

That comment took Ron and me a bit by surprise. I don't know why. We were well aware of the risks for multiple births with my treatment. I guess it took so long to get this far, we couldn't fathom that there could possibly be more than one in there.

We spent that Friday evening visiting our families and sharing the great news. Everyone was _so_ happy and excited. We just couldn't wait to meet the newest member of the family.

I spent the next two weeks agonizing over the possibility that we could have multiples. I wasn't concerned with twin or triplets, and actually I had gotten to the point that I was perfectly fine with anything up to four. It was after four that I got really concerned. The concerns were more related to my health and the babies' health, not so much as the logistics on how to care for them after they got home. I knew that help would probably appear. I knew that there are risks to any multiple birth, but when the number of fetuses is above four, the risks are greatly elevated. So I waited eagerly for the ultrasound on December 16, 1999.

As we visited with Dr. Gold on the day of the ultrasound, she said, "Let's see how many Hansens we have in there." As she inserted the ultrasound wand, she immediately came across a sac. She said, "There it is, sweet baby." She pointed out the yolk sac, the placenta, and the little tiny flicker that was the heartbeat. The whole fetus was only 2 mm, about the size of a grain of rice. The heartbeat was prominent and regular. The sac and placenta looked healthy. I asked how everything looked and she said that what we saw that day was a major step towards a healthy pregnancy. Everything looked very good. Then she said, "We'll call that baby #1." My eyes got really big as she began moving the ultrasound wand around a little bit... and she found no more sacs. I was pregnant with one baby.

Conclusion

The Fork in the Road

The <u>very</u> first ovulation induction cycle with an IUI <u>after</u> lowering my insulin level to 5.3 by altering my eating habits resulted in a successful pregnancy! This is monumental! The insulin discovery changed my life. And I am convinced that it saved my life. I am fully aware now that I am insulin resistant, and it directly effects the severity of my PCOS. This prognosis will be with me *forever*, not just while I am trying to achieve a pregnancy. If I were to continue living life ignoring the dietary requirements that keep my insulin low, my pancreas may some day just run out of insulin. If that were to happen, I would have insulin-dependent diabetes. I would then be subject to major diabetes management and to all of the damage that diabetes can inflict on a body, including cardiovascular disease (CVD), blindness, high blood pressure, blood clotting and stroke. Finding this prognosis out in my thirties probably saved a good twenty years of damage. So, in fact the inability to get pregnant was indeed a blessing, for it led to me this life-altering diagnosis. For this reason, I like to refer to my PCOS in a positive light, leading me to the title "Positively PCOS."

Even though I will need to monitor my diet forever, my doctors advised that I should proceed through the pregnancy with a "normal" diet. What they meant by "normal" was to eat smart and healthy by eating balanced meals, but not by completely restrict the carbs like I had been doing. This would provide the necessary nourishment that the developing baby would need during pregnancy and later, breastfeeding. I was warned that I should return, however, to the lower-carb lifestyle (not no-carb) after breastfeeding, in order to keep a handle on my insulin levels.

Becoming pregnant was absolutely thrilling, *but* I had done so much research on IR and PCOS that I knew I was at great risk for miscarriage[24]. I was therefore referred to a "high risk" fetal/maternal physician. There have been studies done to discover why polycystic ovaries are seen in a large percentage of patients that have suffered miscarriages. There are a few leading conclusions. The first is hyperinsulinemia, in which elevated levels of insulin disturb the normal blood clotting factors, obstructing the interface between the uterine lining and the placenta. The second is elevated LH secretions have been thought to cause chromosomally abnormal eggs. Another study looks at how high androgen levels may also be a contributing factor in egg quality[25]. There is also the possibility of deficient progesterone to support the developing fetus, hence my progesterone oil injections.

---

[24] "Polycystic Ovary Syndrome-Miscarriage and complications of pregnancy in women with and without PCOS" states that women with PCOS have up to a 44% first trimester miscarriage rate.

[25] Perloe, Mark. "Polycystic Ovary Syndrome... Treatment with Insulin Lowering Medications." 26 Aug 1999. <http://www.ivf.com/pcostreat.html>

So instead of rejoicing, I was worried. I anguished over every ping and pang my body felt. *Please don't let me lose this baby.* I prayed and prayed. It was forty very, very long weeks.

I joyfully announce that we had a son on July 29, 2000. He was 6 lbs. 2 oz, 20¼ inches and just the most beautiful creation I had ever laid my eyes on. We were in absolute wonder at the miracle that lay before us. I also happened to have an exceptional birthing experience and am in complete awe of the process. My doctor's office had a certified nurse midwife (CNM) join their practice just about 3 weeks before my due date and since my birthing plan called for "a natural birthing experience" (no drugs), they asked if I would like to meet her. I said, "Sure!", but I honestly didn't think that this would be something for me. When I thought "midwife", my thoughts were about home-births and no facilities available for emergencies. That was until she walked into the room and began talking with me. I loved her! I brought Ron to the next appointment to get his opinion and he was comfortable with her too. With our CNM's assistance, I naturally delivered our son at a hospital (not at home) without the use of an epidural.

This is when I arrived at my new fork in the road. For, when walking this new road, I am a nurturer, caregiver, educator, advocate, mother.

Our dreams and prayers for a family were *finally* answered. It took me three and a half years to get pregnant after I discontinued using birth control pills. The road that Ron and I traveled was by no means a leisurely stroll. It was frustrating, scary, sad, emotionally draining, gratifying, painful, exciting, and exhilarating. But not all at the same time. We have a much bigger appreciation for every gift from God, especially His children. They are the most amazing of His creations. The world seems to be a much different place now. I still live and work in the same environment, but my perspective has changed. The sky is bluer, the birds sing louder, the rain smells refreshing. Did I notice these things before? Maybe a little, but not with the appreciation I have today. Life is good! And it is even better when you have traveled through the darkness to get to light.

Good Luck and God Bless.

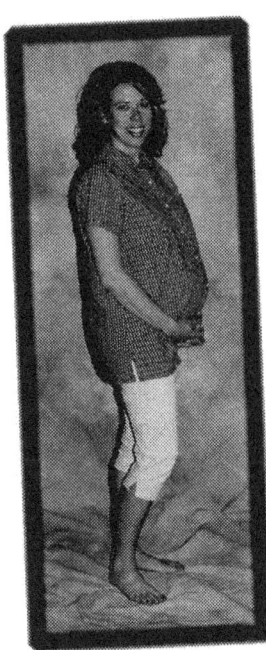

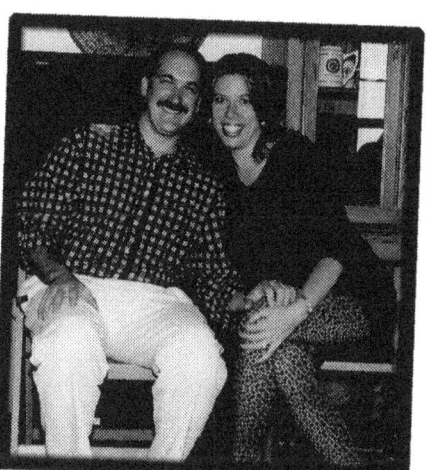

Ron and Amy at baby shower

Amy, 5 days before
Erek was born

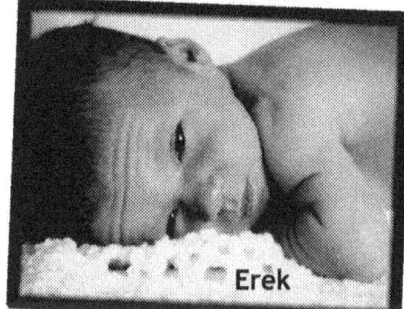

Erek

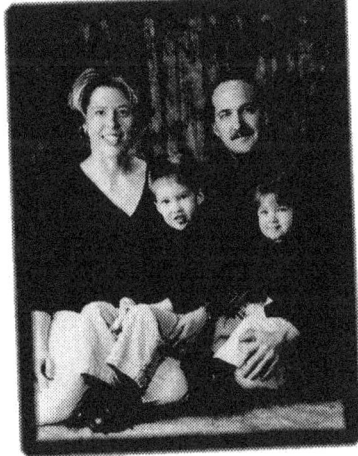

Amy, Ron, Erek and Emma

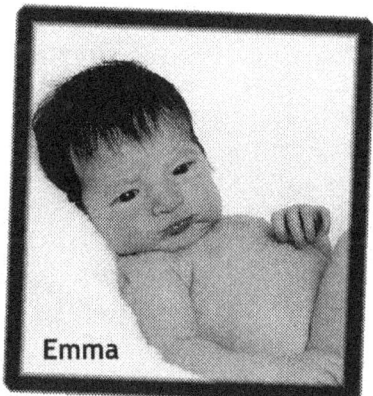

Emma

Final Comments

I have now focused much of my time and research on the effects of IR and its relationship to diabetes. Once I achieved the positive pregnancy results, I wanted to know everything about this condition that had so much control over my hormone levels. Advocacy, publicity, and knowledge will help others become aware of this syndrome.

While we waited for the arrival of our "miracle child", I sometimes reflected in amazement at all that we had endured over the previous three years. And then I had an idea. There must be other people out there that are suffering through the similar, if not same despair that we were. I know how alone and how hurt one can feel. What if I tried to do what I could to raise awareness and advocate education on the disease that controlled my reproductive process? I decided that I could accomplish this by sharing our experience and communicate what we had learned.

Therefore, I began to convert my journal and record-keeping into my story. I wrote most of this story by the time my son was born in 2000, but becoming a new mom completely put everything on hold for a while. I wanted to savor all of the time I had with him. And to our delight, when our son was 11 months old, we were able to conceive another baby with exactly the same amount of medication and IUI as our previous successful attempt. We greeted a daughter into our family on March 22, 2002.

The key to my body is insulin sensitivity. Before we started to try for baby #2, I had a fasting insulin test and the result was 11. I refrained from high sugars and high carbs for six weeks, had another test done and it was only at 10. Better, but not low enough. I went back again after four more weeks and the result was 4.5. The very first ovulation induction cycle attempt for my second child worked. Our children are twenty months apart.

My body still does not generate a menstrual cycle on its own. I induce my cycles four times a year with Provera™. I have to always be conscience of focusing on a healthy balanced diet. I am not on the restricted Atkins' diet. However, I watch my carb intake and try to link-and-balance my foods as I eat. If I eat too much sugar at one time, by body responds accordingly, with a headache. I now take 500mg of Metformin a day and check my fasting insulin levels once a year.

While I compiled my history to write this story, I continued researching the topics of PCOS and IR. During the search for more information, I came across new and exciting publications. One was a book called <u>PCOS: The Hidden Epidemic</u> *by Samuel S. Thatcher, M.D., Ph.D. I have found this to be the single most informative book thus far that covers PCOS entirely, including insulin resistance. I thoroughly enjoyed the reading and refer back to it all of the time for definitions or references. What I like most about it is that it contains more than just surface material on PCOS. I was looking for more in-depth details, and this book is a huge help. I think that it provides invaluable information for the PCOS patient and physician. It was in this book that I found the statement, "PCOS is the most common cause of infertility in women who don't ovulate." If I would have only known then, what I know now.*

*Another fantastic source of information is the Polycystic Ovarian Syndrome Association (PCOSA) at **www.pcosupport.org.** A huge part of battling this syndrome is the community of support with others. The message boards at this website provide such a lifeline of support.*

And now the Internet is such a great source of information. One article called PCOS "the archetypal Internet disease": "Women find out about it from a friend. Then they go to the Internet and read about it." [26]

Finally, in order to help understand dietary requirements for my hyperinsulinemia, I read The Insulin-Resistance Diet by Cheryle R. Hart, M.D. and Mary Kay Grossman, R.D. I highly recommend this book to understand how what we eat effects our blood sugar and insulin production. It describes how to "link-and-balance" food when we eat to minimize a significant change in our blood sugar levels. I found this very insightful.

I have included a page of information on glucose, diabetes and insulin resistance that summarizes terms associated with diabetes and explains what happens after we eat our food for energy. The information comes from a clinical nutrition textbook used by dieticians. I thought the explanations were very clear, easy to understand and very useful.

Now I am going to re-iterate how important it is to read, research and read some more if you believe that you or someone you know is suffering from PCOS, Insulin Resistance or Diabetes. You must make your voice heard and equip yourself with the knowledge to find a doctor that is right for you. Unfortunately, PCOS is so often misdiagnosed and overlooked. In the article "Hide and Seek," the author's doctor, Dr. Samuel Thatcher, MD, Ph.D, states "health care professionals typically either overlook the symptoms or see symptoms as isolated rather than related to one another." The article goes further to say that "women with PCOS often report that they have to see an average of eight to nine physicians before a PCOS diagnosis is made." While the symptoms are blatantly clear to some of us that are living with the syndrome, some physicians have just never heard of PCOS nor Insulin Resistance. According to PCOS: The Hidden Epidemic (p.12), "PCOS is the most common hormonal disorder among pre-menopausal women." The is still a lot of unpredictability and unknown territory with PCOS, but in just a few years time, the information that has been discovered and published has grown leaps and bounds.

I still believe that the largest misunderstanding with Insulin Resistance right now is the Fasting Insulin and Fasting Glucose levels. I know the difference between the two tests but apparently I cannot convince some physicians that the INSULIN test is appropriate for certain patients that exhibit signs and symptoms of Insulin Resistance. Most physicians will only test your fasting insulin IF only

---

[26] Roan, Shari. "When Hormones go Haywire." Well and Healthy Woman magazine. April 2002. 25 Jun 2003. <http://www.whwmag.com/issue/2002/04/staywell/article1.asp>

your fasting glucose comes back elevated, indicating the possibility of diabetes. This is not true in my situation and according to several sources, "Chang studied glucose and insulin levels of normal-weight women with PCOS and found that although their glucose levels were normal, their insulin levels were much higher than those of women without the syndrome,"[27] "insulin resistance may be present in advance of or without elevated glucose levels,"[28] "people with insulin resistance have normal to low glucose levels and higher than normal insulin levels."[29]

And then there is the controversy over what constitutes an elevated fasting insulin level. There has not been standardization on this subject across the medical community. I have seen many different acceptable levels published. Some have stated that 15 uIU/ml constitutes an elevated fasting level, and others will say 10 uIU/ml.[30] Here is what I do know. There are studies that suggest insulin levels effect egg quality, uterine lining quality, and can disturb the normal blood clotting factors, obstructing the interface between the uterine lining and the placenta. I carried two successful pregnancies AFTER my insulin levels were reduced to a level between 4-5 uIU/ml. My insulin levels before dietary changes were over 10 uIU/ml. However, I typically weigh between 140-150 pounds. I am not suggesting that others' insulin levels would mimic mine, but this was a huge factor for me to successfully conceive and carry a child.

And finally, there are other risk factors to be aware of in patients that have been diagnosed with Insulin Resistance. If there is consistent excess insulin made by the body, it can eventually cause Adult Onset Diabetes (Type II). Diabetes promotes atherosclerosis (plaque on artery walls), damage to the inner linings of the artery walls and clot formation (causes strokes). Excessive insulin can also cause the liver to produce a lot of cholesterol (causing high blood cholesterol), cause the blood vessels of the body to be damaged by promoting high blood pressure and tell the body to store fat causing obesity. Damage to the large blood vessels can cause Cardiovascular Disease (CVD) which is the leading cause of death in adult onset diabetes. Furthermore, damage to the small blood vessels can damage the kidneys and cause blindness.

All of this information is not meant to scare or terrify you. It is only meant to educate and inform. I hope that the information has been helpful, informative, and my story slightly entertaining at times. I believe that if this helps just ONE person, then it has served its purpose. A few years back when I was feeling the most vulnerable after treatment, I had questioned my life and its purpose. I kept searching and searching. I just wanted to know what I was here to do, so that I

---

[27]   "Polycystic Ovary Syndrome: Metabolic Challenges and New Treatment Options" Medical Association Communications. 1999. 30 Sep 1999. <http://www. macmcm.com/asrm/asrm98-pos.html>

[28]   PCOS: The Hidden Epidemic p. 77

[29]   The Insulin Resistance Diet p. 18

[30]   PCOS: The Hidden Epidemic *states that "Thin, "normal" women have an average level of about 10; while in obese women the level has increased to 15. Probably levels much under 15 are clearly normal and much over 25 clearly elevated."*

could get working on "it." Maybe it would fulfill what was missing and raise my spirits. But I couldn't figure out what "it" was, and like so many others that are doing the searching, "it" found me.

I know now that my purpose at this time in my life is to advocate and communicate the effects of PCOS and IR, and the prevention of Diabetes. According to the Polycystic Ovarian Syndrome Association, the syndrome affects approximately 5-10 % of all women worldwide, and many are undiagnosed. I truly believe that communication and awareness are necessary to save lives.

When I started publicly sharing my experience openly with others that asked about it, my purpose started to make more sense to me. This was a method of healing for me, and a sense of comfort for others. Comfort in the fact that there may still be hope for them. Many people also become intrigued and eager to learn more. And this is the spark that starts the education flame.

In closing, no matter what your diagnosis is, educate yourself as much as you can on the subject and more. I have found out first-hand that it pays off. You need to be actively participating in the management of your health. Hopefully, you can feel as comfortable with your physician, as I was with mine. I believe that this relationship is very critical in receiving adequate and appropriate care. We've each been given only one lifetime.

Information on glucose, diabetes and insulin resistance

Glucose

The human body needs "fuel" to operate or function properly, just as a car needs fuel to run. The food that we eat is the source of this fuel, and our body responds accordingly. Our bodies convert the food we eat into an energy source called **glucose,** or "blood sugar". Glucose provides about half of the energy that we need for our bodies, and fat provides the other half. We cannot eat glucose directly; we eat foods rich in carbohydrates. Carbohydrates are found in all unrefined plant foods – whole grains, vegetables, legumes, and fruits. They are also found in sugars, honey and milk. Glucose is the simplest sugar and the only one that your body can use for energy.

A certain amount of glucose is needed in the blood in order to function or feel well. If your blood sugar falls below normal, you may feel shaky, tired or hungry. If your blood sugar goes above normal, you may become fatigued. If either extreme is pushed far enough, you go into a coma.

Every cell in your body depends on glucose to an extent. In fact, the brain relies mainly on glucose. As a bonus, your body maintains the blood glucose level for you. When you wake in the morning, your fasting blood glucose level is probably between 70-120 milligrams (mg) of glucose per 100 per milliliters (ml). If you do not eat, your blood glucose level will eventually fall. Most people experience the feeling of being hungry at around 60-65 mg. The response to that is to eat, and the blood sugar rises again.

At the other end of the spectrum, is when the blood sugar levels get too high. Special cells of the pancreas, beta cells, are sensitive to the blood glucose levels. When blood glucose rises, these special cells release a hormone called insulin into the blood. The hormone insulin causes glucose to be withdrawn from the bloodstream and transported to your body cells where it is used for energy. If there is more glucose in the bloodstream than your body needs, the insulin sends it to be stored in the liver and muscle cells as glycogen. The liver also converts some of the extra glucose to be stored as fat. Ultimately, your blood glucose level returns to a normal range, and the excess glucose is stored as glycogen (can return to glucose) and fat (cannot return to glucose).[31]

---

[31]   Whitney, Eleanor, Corinne Balog Cataldo and Sharon Rady Rolfes, Understanding Normal and Clinical Nutrition. Sixth Edition. Belmont, CA: Wadsworth/Thompson Learning, 2002.

Diabetes and Insulin Resistance

"**Diabetes** mellitus is caused by a lack of insulin, a hormone manufactured by the pancreas. Type II diabetes or non-insulin-dependent diabetes (NIDDM), usually occurs in people aged over 40, especially when they are overweight. This is the type of diabetes which women with PCOS are at an increased risk of developing. Some experts suggest the increase is as much as ninefold.

People with type II diabetes have plenty of insulin in the body but their tissues are insensitive to it and don't use it well (a problem called **insulin resistance**). Insulin resistance is linked to a higher risk of developing diabetes type II or NIDDM."[32]

When there is a lack of insulin secreted by the pancreas, it creates a buildup of glucose in the bloodstream called hyperglycemia. High levels of glucose in the blood over a long period of time, affects other parts of the body and can be very damaging. That is why other complications usually come up when people are diagnosed with diabetes.

"Disorders of the large blood vessels, such as coronary heart disease and hypertension, are common in people with diabetes. Cardiovascular disease tends to develop early, progress rapidly, and be more advanced at the time of diagnosis in people with type II diabetes. Disorders of the small blood vessels (capillaries) may also develop, affecting the eyes, kidneys or nervous system. Diabetes affects the structures of blood vessels and nerves, leading to impaired circulation, impaired vision, and loss of sensation in the limbs. Diabetes is the leading cause of both kidney disease and blindness."[33]

If caught early on, type II diabetes can be managed and treated before other complications arise. Managing diabetes means maintaining normal blood glucose levels. Treatment plans can include a new diet plan, physical exercise and possibly medication. Untreated or ignored diabetes type II can result in the inability of the pancreas to create insulin, resulting in Insulin Dependent Diabetes or IDDM. Insulin dependent diabetes requires insulin injections to maintain healthy blood glucose levels.

---

[32] Harris, Colette and Dr. Adam Carey, PCOS A Woman's Guide to Dealing with Polycystic Ovary Syndrome. London: Thorsons, 2000.

[33] Whitney, Eleanor, Corinne Balog Cataldo and Sharon Rady Rolfes, Understanding Normal and Clinical Nutrition. Sixth Edition. Belmont, CA: Wadsworth/Thompson Learning, 2002.

Interesting Quotes

Bender, Ellen Friedman – "New Directions in the Treatment of Polycystic Ovarian Syndrome", November 1999 issue of Women's O.W.N. of NYU Medical Center newsletter www.Americaninfertility.org

> PCOS is being recognized as a major women's health problem because of the havoc it wreaks on the endocrine system. What is significant is that women who have PCOS are seven times more likely to suffer from adult onset diabetes. Additionally, over time, many women with PCOS develop elevated levels of cholesterol and triglycerides so that there is greater risk of heart attack and stroke for women in the forties and fifties. And because of the irregular cycles, women with PCOS are at greater risk for endometrial cancer. Women with PCOS frequently encounter self-esteem and body-image issues because of the symptoms from the disorder including excess facial hair, obesity, acne, male-pattern baldness, and hirsutism.

Medical Association Communications – "Polycystic Ovary Syndrome: Metabolic Challenges and New Treatment Options", October 6, 1998. www.macmcm.com

> Study showed glucose and insulin levels of normal-weight women with PCOS and found that although their glucose levels were normal, their insulin levels were much higher than those of women without the syndrome. Thus, many women with PCOS appear to be Insulin Resistant.

> Insulin Resistance in PCOS is associated with abnormal cellular glucose transport in insulin-responsive tissues, most likely because of post-receptor signaling aberrations. In turn, IR results in compensatory hyperinsulinemia, with the excess insulin causing an exaggerated effect in other less traditionally responsive tissues (e.g., excess androgen secretion by the ovarian theca; excess growth of the basal cells of the skin, resulting in acanthosis nigricans; increased vascular and endothelial reactivity, resulting in hypertension; and abnormal hepatic and peripheral lipid metabolism, leading to dyslipidemia).

> Many women with PCOS have a defect in insulin secretion, not just insulin action. In other words, their pancreas does not secrete insulin properly.

Although Insulin Resistance is not a recognized medical disorder, if IR is the primary defect in PCOS, then we should treat the IR and not the symptoms that result from it.

Treatment of PCOS includes dietary changes, increasing exercise and possibly medication. Whether Metformin is effective in lean women with PCOS is not yet known.

Perloe, Mark - "Polycystic Ovary Syndrome... Treatment with Insulin Lowering Medications" www.ivf.com/pcostreat.html
Most labs report levels less than 25-30 miu/ml as normal, while in fact, levels over 10 miu/ml on a fasting blood sample suggests that PCOS may be related to hyperinsulinism.

Metformin, Glucophage™, Rezulin™ (troglitazone), Avandia™ (rosiglitazone). These medications have been shown to reverse the endocrine abnormalities seen with polycystic ovary syndrome within two or three months. They can result in decreased hair loss, diminished facial and body hair growth, normalization of elevated blood pressure, regulation of menses, weight loss and normal fertility.

Mann, Denise – "New drug treats polycystic ovary syndrome" April 28, 1999 www.pcosupport.org/pcosinfo/treatments.html
PCOS is a general health issue, not just a fertility issue. Women with PCOS are at high risk for diabetes and heart attacks due to high levels of insulin and blood pressure and triglycerides."
"When the body fails to use insulin properly, the amount of insulin in the blood surges, leading to high blood pressure, high triglyceride level, and arterial disease. Insulin may also cause the ovaries to produce high levels of testosterone, which disrupts menstruation and prohibits ovulation.

The Cholesterol Center at The Jewish Hospital. Cincinnati, Ohio Jan 11, 1999 "Polycystic Ovary Syndrome"
Women with PCOS have up to a 44% first trimester miscarriage rate. Speculative causes for this high miscarriage rate include high levels of PAI-1 (blood clotting) high levels of testosterone, androgens and low levels of progesterone.

In aggregate, hyperinsulinism and resultant hyperandrogenism chronically alter gonadotropin secretion, increasing LH, disrupting the normal pituitary-ovarian axis, leading to amenorrhea (absence of menstrual cycles) and infertility. Hyperinsulinism, in conjunction with hyperandrogenemia, also leads to morbid obesity, hirsutism, acne, frequent hypertension (high blood pressure), hyperlipidemia (high cholesterol), and increased levels of PAI-1 (blood clotting factor), which together increase risk for myocardial infarction (heart attack) and stroke later in life. Hyperinsulinemia, independent of other risk factors for coronary heart disease (CHD), is a major CHD risk factor. Insulin resistance-hyperinsulinemia is also risk factor for noninsulin dependent, mature onset diabetes, common in PCOS.

The New England Journal of Medicine. "Insulin and the Polycystic Ovary Syndrome", 08/29/1996
The evidence that insulin directly stimulates ovarian function is stronger than the evidence that is stimulates luteinizing hormone (LH) secretion.

Hyperinsulinemia, therefore, is a key component of the polycystic ovary syndrome. It is caused by insulin resistance – more specifically, resistance to the hypoglycemic actions of insulin.

PCOS: The Hidden Epidemic, Thatcher, Samuel S., M.D., PhD.
Pg. 74. Not all PCOS patients, especially those with high insulin levels, have an elevation in LH. In fact, PCOS patients that have normal LH levels may be more likely to fall into the high insulin group, or high adrenal hormone group.

Pg 77. Insulin resistance may be present in advance of or without elevated glucose levels. Insulin levels should be obtained fasting and possibly after a glucose challenge. What constitutes a normal insulin level has not been satisfactorily determined. Usually levels above 20 are associated with IR and levels under 10 are considered normal.

Pg 152. Insulin may directly interfere with normal follicle development by indirectly increasing ovarian androgens or by disturbing gonadotropin release from the pituitary gland. Androgens are known to arrest normal development of ovarian follicles and cause their degeneration. LH is known to stimulate the proliferation of androgen producing cells in the theca lay of the ovary. *Any action that can increase androgens or LH can cause PCOS. Insulin may do both.*

Pg 153. Fasting insulin levels. Thin, "normal" women have an average level of about 10; while in obese women the level has increased to 15. It depends on how discriminating one wants to be with the test. Probably levels much under 15 are clearly normal and much over 25 clearly elevated.

Roan, Shari – "When Hormones go Haywire", <u>Well and Healthy Woman magazine</u>

A University of Chicago study found that one in 10 women with PCOS will develop diabetes by age 40. And a 1998 Australian study estimated that PCOS patients have a 7.4 times greater risk of heart attack.

This is the archetypal Internet disease. Women find out about it from a friend. Then they go to the Internet and read about it.

<u>The Insulin Resistance Diet,</u> Hart, Cheryle R., M.D. and Grossman, Mary Kay, R.D.

Pg. 18. You can have Insulin Resistance, however, even with very normal blood glucose levels. A fasting insulin blood level that is higher than 10 iUI/ml is also a flag for insulin resistance. People with insulin resistance have normal to low glucose levels and higher than normal insulin levels.

Appendix A

Homemade Hormone Chart

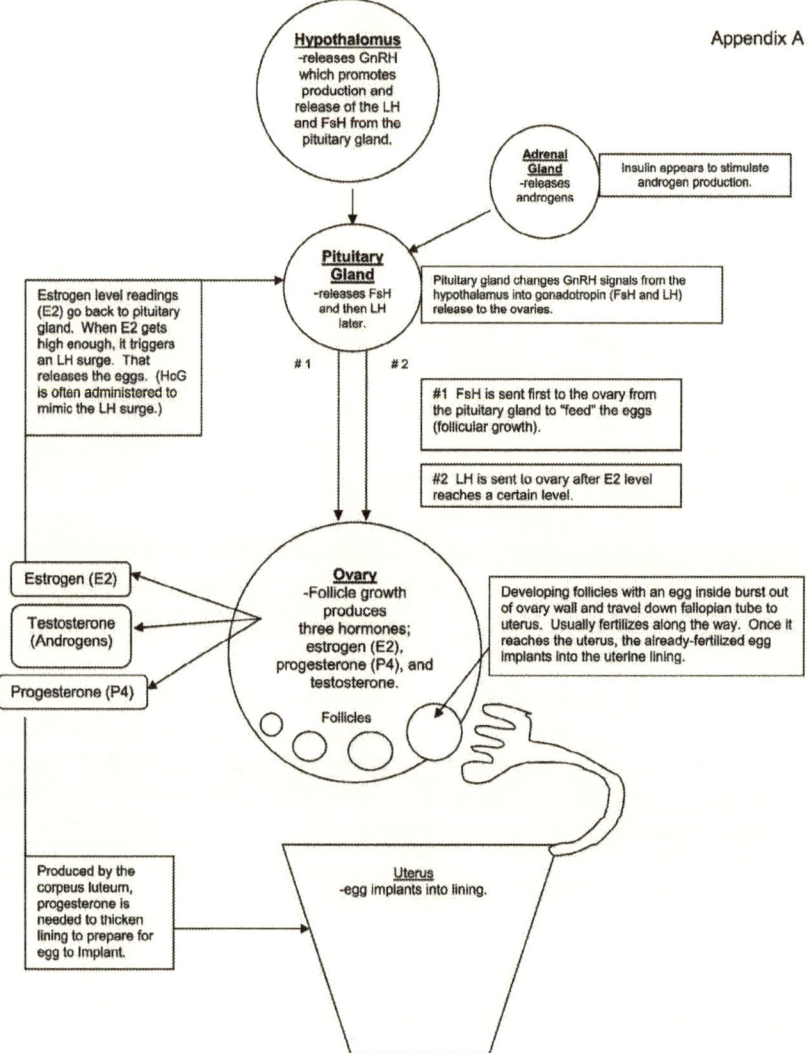

Hypothalomus
-releases GnRH which promotes production and release of the LH and FsH from the pituitary gland.

Adrenal Gland
-releases androgens

Insulin appears to stimulate androgen production.

Pituitary Gland
-releases FsH and then LH later.

Pituitary gland changes GnRH signals from the hypothalamus into gonadotropin (FsH and LH) release to the ovaries.

Estrogen level readings (E2) go back to pituitary gland. When E2 gets high enough, it triggers an LH surge. That releases the eggs. (HcG is often administered to mimic the LH surge.)

1   # 2

#1 FsH is sent first to the ovary from the pituitary gland to "feed" the eggs (follicular growth).

#2 LH is sent to ovary after E2 level reaches a certain level.

Estrogen (E2)

Testosterone (Androgens)

Progesterone (P4)

Ovary
-Follicle growth produces three hormones; estrogen (E2), progesterone (P4), and testosterone.

Follicles

Developing follicles with an egg inside burst out of ovary wall and travel down fallopian tube to uterus. Usually fertilizes along the way. Once it reaches the uterus, the already-fertilized egg implants into the uterine lining.

Produced by the corpeus luteum, progesterone is needed to thicken lining to prepare for egg to implant.

Uterus
-egg implants into lining.

In reality, the uterus is about the size of a pear.

Appendix B

MedicalLog

MEDICAL LOG

Date	Event	Description	Notes	Meds	Cycle Day	Beta Subunit	Estrodial	Insulin (0-21)	Glucose (65-110)
8-Sep-99	Bloodwork	Weight 150		Lupron	Cycle 2		57		
9-Sep-99	Bloodwork			Lupron	Cycle 3			5.3	82
10-Sep-99				Lupron	Cycle 4				
11-Sep-99				Lupron	Cycle 5				
12-Sep-99				Lupron	Cycle 6				
13-Sep-99		Weight 145		Lupron	Cycle 7				
14-Sep-99		Weight 145		Lupron	Cycle 8				
15-Sep-99				Lupron, 2mg Estrace	Cycle 9		43		
16-Sep-99				Lupron, 2mg Estrace	Cycle 10				
17-Sep-99				Lupron, 2mg Estrace	Cycle 11				
18-Sep-99		Weight 146		Lupron, 2mg Estrace	Cycle 12				
19-Sep-99				Lupron, 2mg Estrace	Cycle 13				
20-Sep-99				Lupron, 2mg Estrace	Cycle 14				
21-Sep-99		Weight 147		Lupron, 2mg Estrace	Cycle 15				
22-Sep-99		Weight 149		Lupron, 6mg Estrace	Cycle 16				
23-Sep-99				Lupron, 6mg Estrace	Cycle 17				
24-Sep-99	Ultrasound	Lining at 7mm Add 8mg Estrogen Patches		Lupron, 6mg Estrace	Cycle 18				
25-Sep-99				Lupron, 6mg Estrace, Estrogen patches	Cycle 19				
26-Sep-99				Lupron, 6mg Estrace, Estrogen patches	Cycle 20				
27-Sep-99				Lupron, 6mg Estrace, Estrogen patches	Cycle 21				
28-Sep-99	Ultrasound	Weight 146-7		Lupron, 6mg Estrace, Estrogen patches	Cycle 22				
29-Sep-99		Lining at 13mm		Lupron, 6mg Estrace, Estrogen patches	Cycle 23				
30-Sep-99				6mg Estrace, 6mg Estrogen patches	Cycle 24				
1-Oct-99	FET			6 mg Estrace, 2cc Prog Oil, 1 pre-natal vitamin	Cycle 25				
2-Oct-99				6 mg Estrace, 2cc Prog Oil, 1 pre-natal vitamin	Cycle 26				
3-Oct-99				6 mg Estrace, 2cc Prog Oil, 1 pre-natal vitamin	Cycle 27				
4-Oct-99				6 mg Estrace, 2cc Prog Oil, 1 pre-natal vitamin	Cycle 28				
5-Oct-99				6 mg Estrace, 2cc Prog Oil, 1 pre-natal vitamin	Cycle 29				
6-Oct-99				6 mg Estrace, 2cc Prog Oil, 1 pre-natal vitamin	Cycle 30				
7-Oct-99				6 mg Estrace, 2cc Prog Oil, 1 pre-natal vitamin	Cycle 31				
8-Oct-99				6 mg Estrace, 2cc Prog Oil, 1 pre-natal vitamin	Cycle 32				
9-Oct-99				6 mg Estrace, 2cc Prog Oil, 1 pre-natal vitamin	Cycle 33				
10-Oct-99				6 mg Estrace, 2cc Prog Oil, 1 pre-natal vitamin	Cycle 34				
11-Oct-99		Weight 145		6 mg Estrace, 2cc Prog Oil, 1 pre-natal vitamin	Cycle 35				
12-Oct-99				6 mg Estrace, 2cc Prog Oil, 1 pre-natal vitamin	Cycle 36				
13-Oct-99				6 mg Estrace, 2cc Prog Oil, 1 pre-natal vitamin	Cycle 37				
14-Oct-99				6 mg Estrace, 2cc Prog Oil, 1 pre-natal vitamin	Cycle 38				
15-Oct-99	Bloodwork			.2cc Lupron	Cycle 39	0			
16-Oct-99				.2cc Lupron	Cycle 40				
17-Oct-99				2cc Lupron	Cycle 41				
18-Oct-99				2cc Lupron	Cycle 42				

Date	Notes	Observations	Medication	Procedure	Cycle	Value
19-Oct-99			2cc Lupron		Cycle 43	
20-Oct-99			2cc Lupron		Cycle 1	
21-Oct-99			2cc Lupron		Cycle 2	
22-Oct-99			2cc Lupron		Cycle 3	
23-Oct-99			2cc Lupron		Cycle 4	
24-Oct-99			2cc Lupron		Cycle 5	
25-Oct-99			2cc Lupron		Cycle 6	
26-Oct-99			2cc Lupron		Cycle 7	
27-Oct-99			2cc Lupron		Cycle 8	
28-Oct-99			2cc Lupron		Cycle 9	
29-Oct-99	HsG and bloodwork	Tubes are clear	2cc Lupron		Cycle 10	10
30-Oct-99			2cc Lupron, 3amps Follistim		Cycle 11	
31-Oct-99			2cc Lupron, 3amps Follistim		Cycle 12	
1-Nov-99			2cc Lupron, 3amps Follistim		Cycle 13	
2-Nov-99		Weight 141	2cc Lupron, 3amps Follistim		Cycle 14	
3-Nov-99			2cc Lupron, 3amps Follistim		Cycle 15	
4-Nov-99			2cc Lupron, 2.5 amps Follistim		Cycle 16	
5-Nov-99			2cc Lupron, 2.5 amps Follistim		Cycle 17	
6-Nov-99	Ultrasound; bloodwork	Several cysts L&R 12-16	2cc Lupron, 2.5 amps Follistim		Cycle 18	1166
7-Nov-99		Weight 140	2cc Lupron, 2.5 amps Follistim		Cycle 19	
8-Nov-99	Ultrasound; bloodwork	Several cysts L&R 14-18	2cc Lupron, 2.5 amps Follistim		Cycle 20	2863
9-Nov-99		Weight 141	2cc Lupron, 2amps Follistim		Cycle 21	
10-Nov-99		Weight 142	2cc Lupron	COAST	Cycle 22	5236
11-Nov-99		Weight 145	2cc Lupron	COAST	Cycle 23	9240
12-Nov-99	Ultrasound; bloodwork		2cc Lupron	COAST; Lab s	Cycle 24	6252
13-Nov-99					Cycle 25	
14-Nov-99	Intrauterine Insemination				Cycle 26	
15-Nov-99			Progesterone Oil		Cycle 27	
16-Nov-99	Hyperstimulation	Weight 147	Progesterone Oil		Cycle 28	
17-Nov-99	Hyperstimulation	Drained 2100 cc from belly	Progesterone Oil		Cycle 29	
18-Nov-99	Hyperstimulation	Drained 1100 cc from belly	Progesterone Oil		Cycle 30	
19-Nov-99	Hyperstimulation	Weight 152.5	Progesterone Oil		Cycle 31	
20-Nov-99	Hyperstimulation	Weight 157	Progesterone Oil		Cycle 32	
21-Nov-99	Hyperstimulation		Progesterone Oil		Cycle 33	
22-Nov-99		Weight 153	Progesterone Oil		Cycle 34	
23-Nov-99		Weight 146	Progesterone Oil		Cycle 35	
24-Nov-99		Weight 143	Progesterone Oil		Cycle 36	
25-Nov-99		Weight 140	Progesterone Oil		Cycle 37	
26-Nov-99		Weight 136	Progesterone Oil		Cycle 38	
27-Nov-99			Progesterone Oil		Cycle 39	
28-Nov-99			Progesterone Oil		Cycle 40	
29-Nov-99		Weight 136	Progesterone Oil		Cycle 41	84
30-Nov-99		Weight 137	Progesterone Oil			
1-Dec-99			Progesterone Oil			143
2-Dec-99		Weight 137	Progesterone Oil			
3-Dec-99		Weight 136	Progesterone Oil			269

106

Appendix C

BBT Charts

Appendix C

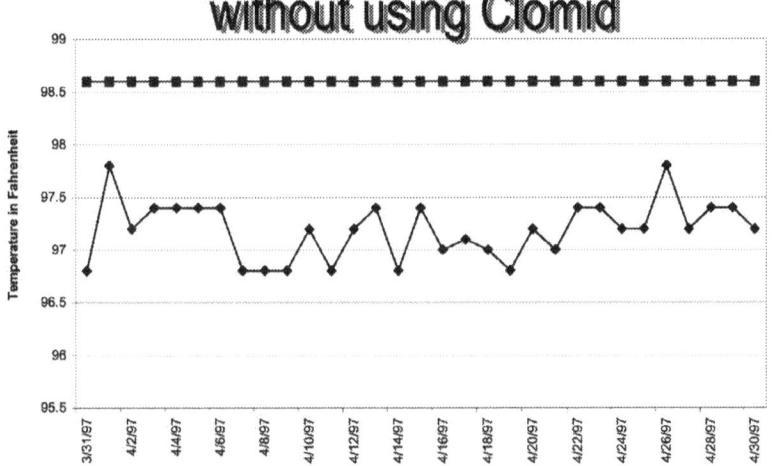

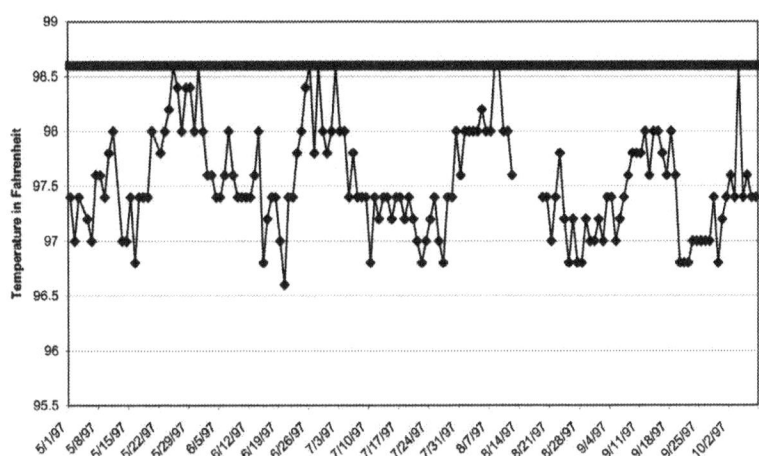

Appendix D

Websites from Page 62

- www.inciid.org (wonderful bulletin boards, helpful glossary),
- www.ivf.com (gives in depth info on IVF, sample pictures),
- www.pcosupport.org (supports PCOS specifically, has message boards),
- www.resolve.org (covers all infertility)

Appendix E

Letter to insurance company

September 10, 1999

Dear XX. XXX,

I am submitting an appeal for the denial of benefits under XXX Plan for the refusal to cover medical treatment regarding infertility.

I was diagnosed in 1996 as Infertile under the definition of Infertility as follows,

> **"Infertility (IF)** -- The inability to conceive after a year of unprotected intercourse in women under 35, or after six months in women over 35, or the inability to carry a pregnancy to term. Also included are diagnosed problems such as anovulation, tubal blockage, low sperm count, etc." (INCIID Web page: http://www.inciid.org/glossary.html).

I will reference the entire clause for infertility coverage as stated in our XXXXX plan document, *"Covered services and supplies solely to diagnose and treat the underlying disease causing Infertility. These services or supplies do NOT include those furnished in order to effect a pregnancy by extraordinary means. (Services and supplies NOT covered include, but are not limited to, Artificial Insemination (AI), In-Vitro Fertilization (IVF), Gamete Intra Fallopian Transfer (GIFT), and Zygote Intra Fallopian Transfer (ZIFT).) These are symptoms that bypass the symptom of Infertility and do not treat the underlying disease condition."*

Under the same plan, I will state services that are exclusively Not Covered, "Number 12 – *A service or supply furnished in order to effect a pregnancy by extraordinary means. These services and supplies include, but are not limited to, Artificial Insemination (AI), In-Vitro Fertilization (IVF), Gamete Intra Fallopian Transfer (GIFT), and Zygote Intra Fallopian Transfer (ZIFT). These are some services that bypass the symptom of Infertility and do not treat the underlying disease condition.*

109

After reviewing the benefits provided under the XXXXX plan, I took note that the *"...services to diagnose and treat the underlying disease causing Infertility..."* were to be covered. I proceeded treatment with a Reproductive Endocrinologist (RE). In fact, the blood work, medication and ultrasounds that were performed to diagnose the inability to conceive, were covered by XXXXX as disclosed. While under the care of Dr. XXX XXX, it was determined through diagnostic treatment that the condition that is preventing conception is PolyCystic Ovarian Syndrome (PCOS), or "Stein-Leventhal Syndrome".

PCOS is defined as "A condition found in women who don't ovulate, characterized by excessive production of <u>androgens</u> and the presence of cysts in the ovaries." The central, probably heritable, biochemical abnormality of polycystic ovary syndrome is hyperinsulinemia. Hyperinsulinemia is the overproduction of insulin that leads to abnormally elevated levels of testosterone and luteinizing hormone (LH). These elevated levels in turn affect the pituitary-ovarian axis, leading to abnormal production of LH and FSH (which stimulate the ovaries). The result of LH and FSH abnormalities is ovarian underproduction of estrogen, along with abnormal production of progesterone, overproduction of testosterone, and amenorrhea and infertility. Hyperinsulinemia has also been associated with high blood pressure and increased clot formation and appears to be a major risk factor for the development of heart disease, stroke and type II diabetes.

What does this mean for PCOS patients that wish to seek treatment to achieve pregnancy? The editorial in "The New England Journal of Medicine" dated August 29, 1996 by Dr Robert D. Utiger, studies the effects of Insulin and PolyCystic Ovary Syndrome.

> *Dr. Utiger summarizes with the question, "What do these new results mean with respect to the treatment of women with the polycystic ovary syndrome? Currently, treatment consists of weight reduction for women who are obese. For those who wish to conceive, clomiphene may be given; if that is unsuccessful, assisted-reproduction procedures or partial ovarian resection may be tried."*

I am considered normal weight and have tried seven clomiphene cycles. The medical industry's recommended number of attempts with clomiphene is six. The XXXXX medical plan states to "... *treat the underlying disease causing Infertility...*". After twenty-one cycle attempts in three years to treat the prognosis of PCOS through medication, I continued to achieve negative results, i.e. low beta results on blood test. While <u>most</u> PCOS patients can achieve pregnancy with medication and vaginal ultrasonic monitoring, there are some cases that require additional medical assistance. We were recommended by our RE that In-vitro Fertilization may increase our chances of conception and be an alternative solution.

As you can see, we have not rushed into our treatment decision with our doctor without due respect for the definition of what is medically necessary. The definition of medically necessary states, "...The service or supply must be consistent with the insured person's medical condition at the time the service is rendered, and is not provided primarily for the convenience of the insured persons doctor..."

I now question the XXXXX plan's exclusion to Assisted Reproduction Technologies (ART), i.e. AI, IVF, GIFT, ZIFT. I am going to explain why XXXXX should include FULL infertility treatment in the plan.

I will first point out that Infertility is a disease. Infertility is a medically recognized disease that is experienced by 6.1 million women and their partners. It is considered a disease by the following organizations.

1. <u>American Society for Reproductive Medicine</u> – "Infertility is a <u>disease</u> of the reproductive system that affects the male or female with almost equal frequency." (ASRM Web page: http://www.asrm.org/fact/infertility.html).
2. <u>Resolve</u> – "Infertility is a <u>disease</u> or condition of the reproductive system." (Resolve Web page: http://www.resolve.org).
3. <u>Numerous health-related organizations</u> – "Infertility is a <u>disease</u> or condition of the reproductive system resulting

in the inability to conceive after one year of unprotected well-timed intercourse. Infertility also includes the inability to carry a pregnancy to the delivery of a live baby." (Web page: http://www.dejanews.com/[tr=altfaz]/article/339989053 - Page 2 of 9; Web page: http://www.fbsims.com/dictionary.html; Web page: http://www.healthatoz.com/alert0298.html).

The Insurance Disease Codebook lists infertility as a disease, and the code for female infertility listed in the Medicode ICD-9 booklet is 628.8. If infertility is not a sickness, why is it listed in this reference book?

In review of the above, the XXXXX plan CANNOT state that infertility is not an illness, and that treatment of infertility is not medically necessary. According to the American Medical Association, the full definition of medical necessity is "*...the shortest, or least intensive level of treatment, care of service rendered, or supply provided, as determined to the extent required to diagnose or TREAT AN INJURY OR SICKNESS. The service or supply must be consistent with the insured person's medical condition at the time the service is rendered, and is not provided primarily for the convenience of the insured persons doctor...*" It would appear that any insurance company's contention that infertility is not an illness or sickness is arbitrary and without foundation.

I'd like to point out that the XXXXX plan provides full coverage for Maternity and Obstetric care; including prenatal and high-risk obstetrical services. Excluding procedures related to the treatment of infertility while covering all other procedures related to reproduction is discriminatory, as it denies those with this disability and medical condition relating to pregnancy access to the medical care necessary for them to engage in the major life activity of reproduction.

The Americans with Disabilities Act (ADA), which was passed in 1991, provides that, it is unlawful to discriminate against persons with disabilities. To be disabled under the ADA, a person must have

"...a physical or mental impairment that substantially limits one or more major life activities..."

According to the Code of Federal Regulations, a physical or mental impairment is defined as, "any physiological disorder, or condition, cosmetic disfigurement, or anatomical loss affecting one or more of the following body systems: Neurological, muscoskelital, special sense organs, respiratory (including speech organs), cardiovascular, **REPRODUCTIVE**, digestive, genital-urinary, hemic and lymphatic, skin, and endocrine..."

The United States Supreme Court ruled in Abbott v. Bragdon, that reproduction is a major life activity. The plaintiff Abbott, a woman who is HIV positive, sued Bragdon, a dentist who refused to treat her in his office because of her HIV status, claiming he discriminated against her under the ADA.

Upon Bragdon's first defeat, he appealed to the circuit court and the circuit court also agreed with Abbott; the 1st Circuit Court of Appeals ruled that asymptomatic HIV positive status was a disability due to the limitations placed on procreation. The following quotation summarizes the Abbott court's decision:

> "The question of whether reproduction in large constitutes a major life activity under the ADA is not free from doubt. The ADA itself does not define the term 'major life activities,' and the few available judicial precedents reveal divergent opinions. Compare Pacourek v. Inland Steel Co., 916 F. Supp. 797, 804 (N.D. Ill. 1996) (finding that reproduction is a major life activity) and Erickson v. Board of Govs. of State Colleges, 911 F. Supp. 316, 323 (N.D. Ill. 1995) (same) and Cain v. Hyatt, 734 F. Supp. 671, 679 (E.D. Pa. 1990) (same) with Krauel v. Iowa Methodist Med. Ctr., 95 F.3d 674, 677 (8th Cir. 1996) (holding that reproduction is not a major life activity) and Zatarain v. WDSU-TV, Inc., 881 F. Supp. 240, 243 (E.D. La. 1995) (same). Still, it is clear that Ms. Abbott's HIV-positive status has a profound impact upon her ability to engage in intimate sexual activity, gestation, giving birth, childrearing, and nurturing familial relations. Our society has long recognized the fundamental importance of each element of this cluster of activities, and our jurisprudence reflects this bias. See, e.g., Stanley v. Illinois, 405 U.S. 645, 651 (1972) **(terming the rights to conceive and raise children 'essential,' 'basic civil rights,' and rights that are 'far more precious . . . than property rights')** (citations and internal quotation marks omitted). Viewed against this backdrop, we think it is highly likely that Congress accorded

113

comparable importance to these activities when it authored the ADA."

Bragdon appealed to the Supreme Court and lost. The following text is from the US Supreme Court's decision.

"**From the outset, however, the case has been treated as one in which reproduction was the major life activity limited by the impairment**. It is our practice to decide cases on the grounds raised and considered in the Court of Appeals and included in the question on which we granted certiorari. See, e.g., Blessing v. Freestone, 520 U.S. 329, 340, n. 3 (1997) (citing this Court's Rule 14.1(a)); Capitol Square Review and Advisory Bd. v. Pinette, 515 U.S. 753, 760 (1995). **We ask, then, whether reproduction is a major life activity**.

We have little difficulty concluding that it is. As the Court of Appeals held, '[t]he plain meaning of the word 'major' denotes comparative importance' and 'suggest[s] that the touchstone for determining an activity's inclusion under the statutory rubric is its significance.' 107 F. 3d, at 939, 940. Reproduction falls well within the phrase 'major life activity.' Reproduction and the sexual dynamics surrounding it are central to the life process itself.

While petitioner concedes the importance of reproduction, he claims that Congress intended the ADA only to cover those aspects of a person's life which have a public, economic, or daily character. Brief for Petitioner 14, 28, 30, 31; see also id., at 36-37 (citing Krauel v. Iowa Methodist Medical Center, 95 F. 3d 674, 677 (CA8 1996)). The argument founders on the statutory language. Nothing in the definition suggests that activities without a public, economic, or daily dimension may somehow be regarded as so unimportant or insignificant as to fall outside the meaning of the word 'major.' The breadth of the term confounds the attempt to limit its construction in this manner.

As we have noted, the ADA must be construed to be consistent with regulations issued to implement the Rehabilitation Act. See 42 U.S.C. _ 12201(a). Rather than enunciating a general principle for determining what is and is not a major life activity, the Rehabilitation Act regulations instead provide a representative list, defining term to include 'functions such as caring for one's self, performing manual tasks, walking, seeing, hearing, speaking, breathing, learning, and working.' 45 CFR _84.3(j)(2)(ii) (1997); 28 CFR _41.31(b)(2) (1997). As the use of the term 'such as' confirms, the list is illustrative, not exhaustive.

These regulations are contrary to petitioner's attempt to limit the meaning of the term 'major' to public activities. The inclusion of activities such as caring for one's self and performing manual tasks belies the suggestion that a task must have a public or economic character in order to be a major life activity for purposes of the ADA. On the contrary, the Rehabilitation Act regulations support the inclusion of reproduction as a major life activity, since reproduction could not be regarded as any less important than working and learning. Petitioner advances no credible basis for confining major life activities to those with a public, economic, or daily aspect. **In the absence of any reason to reach a contrary conclusion, we agree with the Court of Appeals' determination that reproduction is a major life activity for the purposes of the ADA."**

The United State Supreme Court has recognized reproduction as a major life act under the ADA. In summary, the disease of infertility is an impairment that substantially limits the major life activity of reproduction. Thus, infertility is a disability. It is unlawful under the ADA to treat persons with disabilities differently than other employees in the terms or conditions of employment, including fringe benefits.

Title VII of the Civil Rights Act provides that sex discrimination includes discrimination based on pregnancy, childbirth or related medical conditions. It has been held that infertility is a medical condition related to pregnancy. Therefore, an employer cannot treat you any differently than its other employees as far as providing insurance benefits, time off from work, etc. The advantage of the Pregnancy Discrimination Act (PDA) over the ADA is that there is no provision relating to insurance under the PDA. Thus, the costs of providing the coverage are irrelevant, the law simply prohibits discrimination in the terms or conditions of employment, including fringe benefits.

Although the ADA has a specific section, which protects some insurance plans, the Equal Employment Opportunity Commission

(EEOC) has issued guidelines in interpreting this provision. The Guidelines provide that in order to have the protections of the insurance provision for a disability-based distinction, the insurer must establish that it is financially impossible to establish this.

Studies on the cost of infertility coverage have clearly shown that the costs are minimal. Current data suggest that the total cost for covering all aspect of infertility services is approximately $2.00 per month per typical family policy, and that most insurance plans already cover diagnostic services and some forms of treatment. The marginal cost to provide equitable infertility insurance coverage would probably be less than $1.00 per month per family. The true cost to achieve equitable coverage may actually be nothing because the treatments that are most often excluded from insurance coverage (such as In-Vitro Fertilization) are cost-effective and save money relative to surgical treatments that are usually covered within existing policies. It should also be noted that while IVF and related high-tech treatments get the most publicity, the American Society for Reproductive Medicine (ASRM) points out that these technologies account for less than 5 percent of infertility services rendered in the United States.

As indicated earlier, XXXXX coverage does include High-Risk Obstetrics care. The plan document defines this coverage for those women who, *"...have had prior premature infants or miscarriages, or are older first time mothers, or have a CONFIRMED MEDICAL RISK of not being able to carry a baby to term..."* The mere definition to the disease of Infertility states, "...the inability to carry to term" or "...the inability to carry a pregnancy to the delivery of a live baby". Secondly, the conditions of PCOS are proven to make it more difficult to carry a child to term. The miscarriage rate for patients with PCOS is 44% in the first trimester. One of the effects of hyperinsulinemia listed earlier was "increased clot formation" which hinders the quality of the uterine lining for the implantation of the embryo. The diagnosis of PCOS caused by the effects of hyperinsulinemia states that I am at "confirmed medical risk" of not being able to carry a baby to term. Therefore, these treatment measures could be logically added as a service under the High-Risk Obstetrics coverage.

I would not recommend that insurance companies cover endless infertility treatment, yet there are many infertile couples whose chances are cut short due to limited access to insurance coverage. Insurance should be mandated to cover the cost of infertility diagnosis, treatment for the diagnosis and treatment for a certain number of cycles with the reproductive endocrinologist's recommended techniques. Otherwise, set a financial limit to coverage, such as $25,000 specifically for infertility, as some insurance companies do now. Studies show that it takes three procedure attempts on average to achieve success. As I have described above, reproduction is a major life activity that should not be dismissed as "...not medically necessary" or "...not an illness". There should be sufficient medical assistance provided when and if necessary. And in my case, it has been deemed as medically necessary.

In conclusion, I am certain once you examine this grievance, you will conclude, as have I, that XXXXX's denial of coverage for ALL Assisted Reproductive Technologies is out of date and open for litigation, by violating the ADA.

At this point, we are continuing treatment with Dr. XXXX. The IVF procedure that was completed in April provided a successful retrieval of thirty-seven eggs; but the cycle ended with negative pregnancy results. We attempted our first Frozen Embryo Transfer (FET) on June 8th with the embryos attained in the April retrieval, once again with negative pregnancy results. We will again attempt an FET in September 1999, with the embryos attained in the April retrieval.

We fully understand that our physician's policy for each of these procedures is to be paid for in advance and in full, with no guarantee of successful results. The IVF procedure was $4200.00 in total; the physician's fees totaled $1700.00 and the hospital fee was $2500.00. I have attached details and the breakdown of these charges. Each

FET procedure is $779.00 in total; the physician's fee is $360.00 and the hospital fee is $419.00.

I respectfully submit my request to XXXX Corporation to include medically assisted reproduction techniques as an approved medical benefit under the XXXX XXXXX Plan. And therefore, reimbursing the cost of our recent treatments in the total amount of $4979.00. If this is not possible:

◆ I expect a response to my grievance in writing within 30 days or less.

◆ If I am once again denied my claim, I want in writing for XXXXX to "recite, quote and interpret" the "legal" basis reason for my denial.

◆ I want in laymen's terms the clauses and provisions the plan is using for a basis to deny my claim.

◆ I also want to know if XXXXX has ever ruled in favor of a claim in spite of the plan's rules.

◆ Lastly, I need to know if my claim is denied, what my next rights are to appeal and the timetable available to me.

Sincerely,
Amy L. Hansen

cc: Dr. XXXX, Toledo, Ohio
File

Appendix F

Letter response

October 20, 1999

Dear XXX,

I have received the letter ("DBS response letter") from XXX postmarked October 12, 1999 confirming that The Appeals Board for XXXX has denied my appeal for coverage outlined in my September 10, 1999 letter.

The DBS response letter essentially outlines the XXXX section that describes "What's Not Covered" and the right to appeal process. I assume that this is a standard "First Response" letter that follows your appeal process, because my letter clearly stated the same information quoted directly out of the XXXX plan. In other words, we already know what the XXXX plan has outlined as Not Covered. The purpose of my September 10, 1999 appeal letter is to state why our treatment should be covered by XXXX plan.

As stated in the DBS response letter, "At your request we are prepared to treat your September 10th letter as your appeal of this denial and provide you with a full response to that letter", I am requesting that you use my September 10th letter as my written appeal for the denial of medical coverage. The original letter contains my supporting arguments.

Sincerely,

Amy L. Hansen

Summary of Definitions

Unless otherwise noted, the following definitions were gathered from www. inciid.org

Adrenal Glands – releases androgens.

Adrenal Androgens - Male hormones produced by the adrenal gland which, when found in excess, may lead to fertility problems in both men and women. Excess androgens in the woman may lead to the formation of male secondary sex characteristics and the suppression of LH and FSH production by the pituitary gland. Elevated levels of androgens may be found in women with polycystic ovaries, or with a tumor in the pituitary gland, adrenal gland, or ovary. May also be associated with excess prolactin levels.

Amenorrhea – The absence of menstruation. Primary Amenorrhea afflicts a woman who has never menstruated. Secondary Amenorrhea afflicts a woman who has menstruated at one time, but who has not had a period for six months or more.

Androgens - Male sex hormones such as testosterone and DHEAS (Dihydroepiandrosterone Sulfate).

Anovulation - The absence of ovulation.

Artificial Insemination (AI) - Placing sperm into the vagina, uterus or fallopian tubes through artificial means instead of by coitus -- usually injected through a catheter after being washed. This procedure is used for both donor (AID) and husband's (AIH) sperm. This technique is used to overcome sexual performance problems, to circumvent sperm-mucus interaction problems, to maximize the potential for poor semen, and for using donor sperm.

Assisted Reproductive Technology (ART) - Several procedures employed to bring about conception without sexual intercourse, including IUI, IVF, GIFT and ZIFT.

Basal Body Temperature (BBT) - Your body temperature when taken at its lowest point, usually in the morning before getting out of bed. Charting BBT is used to predict ovulation.

Blastocyst –An embryo that has developed for five days after fertilization. At this point theembryo has two different cell types and a central cavity. The surface cells (trophectoderm) will become the placenta, and the inner cell mass, will become the fetus. A healthy blastocyst should hatch from the zona pellucida by the end of the sixth day. Within about 24 hours after hatching, it should begin to implant into the lining of the uterus.

Clomid™ (Brand Name for clomiphene citrate) - Stimulates ovulation through release of gonadotropins (FsH and LH) from pituitary gland. "This medicine is a fertility agent used to stimulate ovulation in women who want to become pregnant. It may also be used to treat other conditions as determined by your doctor." Possible side effects: hot flashes, nausea, vomiting, breast tenderness, dizziness, lightheadedness, headache, or mood changes. Cautions: The medicine may cause dizziness, lightheadedness, or changes in vision. Do not operate machinery, or do anything else that could be dangerous until you know how you react to this medication. Using this medicine may result in multiple pregnancy (twins, etc.). Other brand name: Serophene™ (Description taken from my prescription label)

Corpus Luteum - The yellow-pigmented glandular structure that forms from the ovarian follicle following ovulation. The gland produces progesterone, which is responsible for preparing and supporting the uterine lining for implantation. Progesterone also causes the half-degree or more basal temperature elevation noted after ovulation. If the corpus luteum functions poorly, the uterine lining may not support a pregnancy. If the egg is fertilized, a corpus luteum of pregnancy forms to maintain the endometrial bed and support the implanted embryo. A deficiency in the amount of progesterone produced (or the length of time it is produced) by the corpus luteum can mean the endometrium is unable to sustain a pregnancy. This is called Luteal Phase Defect (LPD).

Crinone™ (Brand name) - a bioadhesive vaginal gel containing micronized progesterone in an emulsion system, which is contained in single use, one piece polyethylene vaginal applicators. Physically, Crinone™ has the appearance of a soft, white to off-white gel. (Description taken from my prescription label)

Cycle day (CD) - The day of a woman's menstrual cycle. The first day (day 1) is when full flow starts before mid-afternoon.

Doxycycline - Antibiotic for reproductive tract. This medicine is a tetracycline antibiotic used to treat bacterial infections. THIS MEDICINE MAY CAUSE increased sensitivity to the sun. Avoid exposure to the sun or sunlamps until you know how you react to this medicine. Use a sunscreen or protective clothing if you must be outside for a prolonged period. IF YOU EXPERIENCE difficulty breathing; tightness of chest; swelling of eyelids, face, or lips; or if you develop a rash or hives, tell your doctor immediately. SIDE EFFECTS, that may go away during treatment, include loss of appetite, nausea, vomiting, or diarrhea. (Description taken from my prescription label)

Embryo - The early products of conception; the undifferentiated beginnings of a baby.

Endometriosis - Growth of endometrial tissue outside the uterus. The tissue may attach itself to the reproductive organs or to other organs in the abdominal cavity. Each month the endometrial tissue inbreeds with the onset of menses. The resultant irritation causes adhesions in the abdominal cavity and in the fallopian tubes. Endometriosis may also interfere with ovulation and with the implantation of the embryo.

Endometrium - The inner lining of the uterus which grows and sheds in response to estrogen and progesterone stimulation; the bed of tissue designed to nourish the implanted embryo.

Estradiol (E2) - The principal estrogen produced by the ovary. Responsible for formation of the female secondary sex characteristics such as large breasts; supports the growth of the follicle and the development of the uterine lining. At mid-cycle the peak estrogen level triggers the release of the LH spike from the pituitary gland. The LH spike is necessary for the release of the ovum from the follicle. Fat cells in both obese men and women can also manufacture estrogen from androgens and interfere with fertility. The blood test to monitor estradiol is E2 -- Rapid Assay. Women on injectible fertility drugs have routine E2 monitoring.

Estriol (E3) – produced by the placenta and is important only in pregnancy. (From PCOS, The Hidden Epidemic. p.73)

Estrogen - The female sex hormones. First recognized around 1915, estrogen is responsible for the development of the secondary feminine sex characteristics, which include breasts, rounded hips, and pubic hair. Together with progesterone, another female hormone made by the ovaries, estrogen regulates the changes that occur with each monthly period and prepares the uterus for pregnancy. See Estradiol.

Estrone (E1) – a weak natural estrogen commonly produced in fat cells; also used in hormone replacement therapy. (From PCOS, The Hidden Epidemic. p.450)

Fallopian Tubes - Ducts through which eggs travel to the uterus once released from the follicle. Sperm normally meet the egg in the fallopian tube, the site at which fertilization usually occurs. The fallopian tube is divided anatomically into a few regions: closest to the uterus and within the uterine wall is the "interstitium" (where interstitial pregnancies develop), next is the "isthmus" (immediately outside the uterine wall) then the "ampulla" (midsection of the tube) and then the "infundibular or fimbrial portion" (adjacent to the ovary at the end of the tube).

Fasting Blood Glucose (FBG) - Blood glucose levels taken after not eating or drinking anything other than water overnight. A normal level is under 110, over 110 shows impaired glucose tolerance or insulin resistance, and over 126 is diabetic. Its ratio in comparison to fasting insulin can also indicate insulin resistance.

Fasting Blood Insulin - Insulin levels taken after not eating or drinking anything other than water overnight. Insulin is a hormone released to break down sugar. Its ratio in comparison to fasting blood glucose can indicate insulin resistance.

Fertinex™ (Brand Name for gonadotropin injectible) - Injectible FsH, subcutaneous. This medicine is a gonadotropin given as an injection for a number of days prior to an injection of human chorionic gonadotropin (hCG) to treat female infertility. SIDE EFFECTS, that may go away during treatment, include abdominal pain or swelling, breast tenderness, or headache. (Description taken from my prescription label)

Follicle - A Fluid-filled sac in the ovary which contains an egg that is released at ovulation. Each month an egg develops inside the ovary in a fluid filled pocket called a follicle. This follicle grows to about one inch in size when it is ready to ovulate.

Follicular Phase – Pre-ovulatory portion of cycle when follicle grows and high levels of estrogen cause the lining to proliferate. Normally between 12-14 days.

Follistim™ (Brand Name for gonadotropin injectible) - Contains human follicle stimulating hormone (FSH). The intrinsic luteinizing hormone (LH) activity in Follistim™ is less that 1 IU per 40,000 IU FSH. The compound is considered to contain no LH activity. Other brand names: Pergonal™, Humegon™, Repronex™, Metrodin™, Fertinex™, Gonal-F™. (Description taken from my prescription label)

Follicle Stimulating Hormone (FsH) - Pituitary hormone that stimulates growth of follicle. Elevated FsH levels are indicative of ovary failure. (Brand names: Follistim™, Fertinex™. Gonal-F™)

Frozen Embryo Transfer (FET) - A procedure where frozen embryos are thawed and then placed into the uterus.

Gonads - The glands that make reproductive cells and "sex" hormones: the testicles, which make sperm and testosterone, and the ovaries, which make eggs (ova) and estrogen.

Gonadotropins - Hormones which control reproductive function: Follicle Stimulating Hormone and Luteinizing Hormone.

Gonadotropin Releasing Hormone (GnRH) - The hormone which controls the production and release of gonadotropins. Secreted by the hypothalamus every ninety minutes or so, this hormone enables the pituitary to secrete LH and FSH, which stimulate the gonads.

Human chorionic gonadotropin (hCG) - The hormone produced in early pregnancy which keeps the corpus luteum producing progesterone. Also used via injection (Profasi™) to trigger ovulation after some fertility treatments, and used in men to stimulate testosterone production. (Brand names: Profasi™, Novarel, Pregnyl)

Human Menopausal Gonadotropins (hMG = Pergonal™, Humegon™, Repronex™) - A combination of hormones FSH and LH, which is extracted from the urine of post-menopausal women. Used to induce ovulation in several fertility treatments.

Home Pregnancy Test (HPT) - A test a woman can use at home to test urine for the presence of hCG.

Hyperglycemia – Elevated blood sugar levels.

Hyperinsulinemia - Overproduction of insulin such as that found in insulin resistance.

Hypoglcemia – A drop in the amount of sugar in the blood.

Hysterosalpingogram (HSG) – and x-ray procedure whereby a special dye is passed through the uterus and tubes to test for structural abnormalities, such as blocked tubes and birth defects of the uterus. (From PCOS, The Hidden Epidemic. p.453)

Infertility - The inability to conceive after a year of unprotected intercourse in women under 35, or after six months in women over 35, or the inability to carry a pregnancy to term. Also included are diagnosed problems such as anovulation, tubal blockage, low sperm count, etc.

Insulin - Hormone used by body to control blood sugar (glucose). IR (overproduction of insulin in relationship to glucose) can lead to weight gain and ovulation difficulties.

Insulin Resistance - Occurs when body produces too much insulin in relation to glucose. One is considered IR with a fasting blood sugar over 110 or a fasting glucose to insulin ratio of less than 4.5:1.

Intra Uterine Insemination (IUI) – A relatively "low-tech" ART which deposits washed sperm directly into the uterus, bypassing cervical mucus and depositing the sperm more closely to the fallopian tubes, where fertilization occurs. Used to bypass hostile cervical mucus and to overcome sperm count and motility problems.

In-vitro Fertilization (IVF) - Literally means "in glass." Fertilization takes place outside the body in a small glass dish.

Luteinizing Hormone (LH) - A pituitary hormone that stimulates the gonads. In the man LH is necessary for spermatogenesis and for the production of testosterone. In the woman LH is necessary for the production of estrogen. When estrogen reaches a critical peak, the pituitary releases a surge of LH (the LH spike), which releases the egg from the follicle.

Lupron™ (Brand name for leuprolide acetate) – Must be refrigerated. Subcutaneous, injectible medication used to down-regulate the pituitary gland and prevent release of substances such as LH and FsH. Without LH and FsH the ovaries will not produce follicles that in turn will decrease Estrogen and Progesterone. This medicine is a gonadotropin-releasing hormone (GnRH) agonist used to treat endometriosis or prostate cancer. It is also used to treat central precocious puberty (CPP). SIDE EFFECTS include hot flashes or sweating; headaches; mood changes; decreased desire for sex; acne; muscle pain or weakness; nausea or vomiting; or changes in breast size. A synthetic nonapeptide analog of naturally occurring gonadotropin releasing hormone (GnRHor IM-RH). It acts as a potent inhibitor of gonadotropin secretion when given continuously and in therapeutic doses. (Description taken from my prescription label)

Luteal Phase – Post-ovulatory phase of a woman's cycle. The corpus luteum produces progesterone, which causes uterine lining to thicken to support the implantation and growth of the embryo.

Metformin (Brand name for metformin hydrochloride) - An insulin altering drug. Metformin is an oral insulin sensitizer that lowers glucose when sugar levels cannot be controlled by diet alone. It enhances the body's sensitivity to insulin and inhibits glucose production from the liver without the risk of hypoglycemia. Other name: Glucophage™. (From PCOS, The Hidden Epidemic. p.371)

Oocyte (Egg, Ovum) – The female reproductive cell.

Ovarian Cyst - A fluid-filled sac inside the ovary. An ovarian cyst may be found in conjunction with ovulation disorders, tumors of the ovary, and endometriosis.

Ovarian Hyperstimulation Syndrome (OHSS) - a syndrome of sudden ovarian enlargement, ascites with or without pain, and/or pleural effusion. A potentially life-threatening side effect of ovulation induction with injectable fertility medications such as hMG and urofollitropins. A woman's ovaries become enlarged and produce an overabundance of eggs. Blood hormone levels rise, fluid may collect in the lungs or abdominal cavity, and ovarian cyst may rupture, causing internal bleeding. Bloodclots sometimes develop. Symptoms include sudden weight gain and abdominal pain. Cycles stimulated with these drugs must be carefully monitored with ultrasound scans. OHSS may be prevented by withholding the hCG injection when ultrasound monitoring indicates that too many follicles have matured. Symptoms are abdominal pain, abdominal distension, gastrointestinal symptoms including nausea, vomiting and diarrhea, sever ovarian enlargement, and weight gain.

Ovary - The female gonad; produces eggs and female hormones.

Ovulation - The release of the egg (ovum, oocyte) from the ovarian follicle.

Ovualtion Induction - use medication to stimulate several follicles to develop on the ovaries.

Pap Smear – Common name of a procedure developed by George Papanicolaou (1883-1962) to detect abnormal cells from the cervix. (From http://cancerweb.ncl. ac.uk)

Paracentesis - The procedure to remove the fluid from the abdominal cavity caused by OHSS. (From PCOS, The Hidden Epidemic. p.382)

Percocet (Brand name oxycodone) - Painkillers. This medicine is an analgesic combination used to relieve pain. SIDE EFFECTS, that may go away during treatment, include dizziness, drowsiness, lightheadedness, constipation, nausea, or vomiting. (Description taken from my prescription label)

Pergonal™ (Brand name) - hMG, Intramuscular FsH. Chemical Name: MENOTROPINS (men-oh-TROE-pins). This medicine is given as an injection for a number of days prior to an injection of human chorionic gonadotropin (hCG) to treat female infertility. It may also be used along with hCG to increase sperm production in men. SIDE EFFECTS, that may go away during treatment, include abdominal pain; fever; chills; muscle or joint pain; skin rash; pain or rash at the injection site; or dizziness. Other brand names: Humegon™, Repronex™. (Description taken from my prescription label)

Pituitary Gland - the master gland, the gland that is stimulated by the hypothalamus and controls hormonal functions. This gland controls major hormonal factories including gonads, thyroid and adrenal glands.

Polycystic – having or involving more than one cyst.

Polycystic Ovary Syndrome - a variable disorder that is marked by amenorrhea, hirsutism, obesity, infertility, and ovarian enlargement and is usually initiated by an elevated level of luteinizing hormone, androgen or estrogen which results in an abnormal cycle of gonadotropins released by the pituitary gland.

Profasi™ (Brand Name) – Human chorionic gonadotropin (HCG), intramuscular injection. Lab Description-Human chorionic gonadotropin (HCG), a polypeptide hormone produced by the human placenta, is composed of an alpha and a beta sub-unit. The alpha sub-unit is essentially identical to the alpha sub-unites of the human pituitary gonadotropins, luteinizing hormone (LH) and follicle-stimulating hormone (FSH), as well as to the alpha sub-unit of human thyroid-stimulating hormone (TSH). Possible side effects: headache, irritability, depression, fatigue, breast tenderness, restlessness, edema. The principal serious adverse reaction during this use are: (1) Ovarian hyperstimulation; (2) Enlargement of preexisting ovarian cysts or rupture of ovarian cysts with resultant hemoperitoneum; (3) Multiple births, and (4) Arterial thromboembolism. Other brand names: Pregnyl, Novarel. (Description taken from my prescription label)

Progestin – a synthetic agent that mimics the action of progesterone. The progestin "matures" the uterine lining and the withdrawal from the medication is what induces a period, as opposed to progesterone which is the hormone naturally produced by the corpus luteum following ovulation to create a lush environment in the uterine lining that is receptive to pregnancy. (From PCOS, The Hidden Epidemic. p.356, 456)

Progesterone (P4) – hormone produced by corpus luteum during second half of cycle. It is released in pulses. Thickens lining. A naturally occurring steroid that is secreted by the ovary, placenta, and adrenal gland. In the presence of adequate estrogen, progesterone transforms a proliferative endometrium into a secretory endometrium. Progesterone is necessary to increase endometrial receptivity for implantation of an embryo. Once an embryo is implanted, progesterone acts to maintain the pregnancy. (Description taken from my prescription label)

Provera™ (Brand name for medroxyprogesterone acetate (MPA)) - Synthetic Progesterone used to treat menstrual disorders. This medicine is used to treat hormonal or menstrual problems. This medicine is a progestin used to treat menstrual disorders. Chemical Name: MEDROXYPROGESTERONE (me-DROX-ee-proe-JESS-te-rone). SIDE EFFECTS that may occur while taking this medicine include nausea, changes in menstrual flow, breakthrough bleeding, spotting, missed periods, breast tenderness, headache, or acne. Other Brand Name: Cycrin™ (Description taken from my prescription label)

Reproductive Endocrinologist (RE) - A medical specialty combining obstetrics and gynecology with endocrinology to treat reproductive disorders.

Testosterone - The male hormone responsible for the formation of secondary sex characteristics and for supporting the sex drive.

Thyroid Gland - The endocrine gland in the front of the neck that produces thyroid hormones to regulate the body's metabolism.

Thyroid Stimulating Hormone (TsH) - Also called thyrotropin. A hormone produced by the pituitary gland (at the base of the brain) that promotes the growth of the thyroid gland (in the neck) and stimulates it.

Transvaginal Ultrasound – A probe (transducer) is inserted into the vagina in order to examine the ovaries and uterus via ultrasound. (From PCOS, The Hidden Epidemic. p.68)

Uterus - The hollow, muscular female reproductive organ that houses and nourishes the fetus during pregnancy. The womb.

Zithromax - Antibiotic to treat bacterial infections. Coordinate with IVF treatment. This medicine is a macrolide antibiotic used to treat bacterial infections. SIDE EFFECTS, that may go away during treatment, include mild diarrhea, nausea, vomiting, or abdominal pain. (Description taken from my prescription label)

Zona Pellucida – Protective coating around the oocyte which protects the oocyte and later, the developing embryo. (From PCOS, The Hidden Epidemic. p.458)

Zygote – Two-cell stage embryo. A fertilized egg which has not yet divided.

Works Cited

Bender, Ellen Friedman. "New Directions in the Treatment of Polycystic Ovarian Syndrome." Women's O.W.N. of NYU Medical Center newsletter November 1999. 01 Feb 2000. <http://www.americaninfertility.org/pcos/aia_benderf.html>

Brody, Jane E. "Syndrome X and Its Dubious Distinction." The New York Times. 10 Oct 2000. Texas Arrhythmia Institute. 4 Sep 2003. <http://www.txai.org/news/2000/00101001.htm>

Combatsyndromex.com 2003. "Insulin Resistance." 4 Sep 2003. <http://www.combatsyndromex.com/insulin.htm>

Glueck, Charles. "Polycystic Ovary Syndrome-Miscarriage and complications of pregnancy in women with and without PCOS." 11 Jan 1999. The Cholesterol Center at The Jewish Hospital, Cincinnati, Ohio. 28 Jul 1999. <http://www.health-alliance.com/hospitals/Jewish/glueck/polycyst.htm>

Hart, Cheryle R., and Mary Kay Grossman, The Insulin Resistance Diet. Chicago: Contemporary Books, 2001

Harris, Collette and Dr. Adam Carey, PCOS A Woman's Guide to Dealing with Polycystic Ovary Syndrome. London: Thorsons, 2000.

INCIID.org. 2000. The InterNational Council on Infertility Information Dissemination, Inc. 12 Apr 2000. <http://www.inciid.org/faq/pcos.html>

Mann, Denise. "New drug treats polycystic ovary syndrome" Reuters Health. New York. April 28, 1999. New England Journal of Medicine. 1999; 340:1314-1320. 30 Jul 1999. <http://www.pcosupport.org/pcosinfo/treatments/html>

Melloni, B. John, Ida G. Dox, Gilbert M. Eisner, June L. Melloni. Melloni's Illutrated Medical Dictionary, Fourth Ed. London: Parthenon Publishing, 2002.

Paolucci, Michelle. "Hide and Seek." NurseWeek Publishing, Inc. 2 Aug 2002. 25 Jun 2003. <http://www.nurseweek.com/news/features/02-08/pcos_print.html>

PCOSupport.org. 1999. Polycystic Ovarian Syndrome Association. 26 Aug 1999. <http://www.pcosupport.org>

Perloe, Mark. "Polycystic Ovary Syndrome... Treatment with Insulin Lowering Medications." 26 Aug 1999. <http://www.ivf.com/pcostreat.html>

"Polycystic Ovary Syndrome: Metabolic Challenges and New Treatment Options" Medical Association Communications. 1999. 30 Sep 1999. <http://www.macmcm.com/asrm/asrm98-pos.html>

Pro-heart.org. Nov 2000. 4 Sep 2003. <http://www.pro-heart.org/s3/site/pdf/RFDiabetesMellitus.pdf>

Roan, Shari. "When Hormones go Haywire." Well and Healthy Woman magazine. April 2002. 25 Jun 2003. <http://www.whwmag.com/issue/2002/04/staywell/article1.asp>

Thatcher, Samuel S., PCOS: The Hidden Epidemic. Indianapolis, Indiana: Perspectives Press, 2000.

The CancerWEB Project. 1997-2003. Dept. of Medical Oncology, University of Newcastle upon Tyne. Medical Dictionary. 12 Sep 2003. <http://cancerweb.ncl.ac.uk>

Utiger, Robert D. "Insulin and the Polycystic Ovary Syndrome." Editorial. The New England Journal of Medicine. 29 Aug 1996. Vol. 335, No. 9. Pg.657-658. 30 Jul 1999. <http://www.nejm.org/content/1996/0335/0009/0657.asp>

Whitney, Eleanor, Corinne Balog Cataldo and Sharon Rady Rolfes. Understanding Normal and Clinical Nutrition. Sixth Edition. Belmont, CA: Wadsworth/Thompson Learning, 2002.

Zouves, Christo, with Julie Sullivan. Expecting Miracles. Henry Holt & Company, Inc., September 15, 1999

Pro-heart.org. Nov 2000. 4 Sep 2003. http://www.pro-heart.org/s3/site/pdf/RFDiabetesMellitus.pdf

About The Author

Amy Hansen lives in a small country town in Ohio with her husband, Ron, and their children, Erek and Emma. She has a degree in finance and worked for a Fortune 500 company for thirteen years, leaving in 2002. She is now a stay-at-home mom whose hobbies include gardening and reading. Amy is also a talented photographer. She continues to pursue the growth of her photography business.

Amy is a member of Polycystic Ovarian Syndrome Association, Inc. (PCOSA) and continues to spread the word about PCOS and insulin resistance. She wants attention to be brought to this often misdiagnosed and under-treated syndrome that affects millions women.

www.ingramcontent.com/pod-product-compliance
Lightning Source LLC
Chambersburg PA
CBHW020442290526
45785CB00002B/967